Intermittent Fasting for Women over 50

The Ultimate Weight Loss Guide to Burn Fat, Slow Aging, Balance Hormones and Live Longer

By Marcy Malone

T he following Book is reproduced below with the goal of providing information that is as accurate and reliable as possible. Regardless, purchasing this Book can be seen as consent to the fact that both the publisher and the author of this book are in no way experts on the topics discussed within and that any recommendations or suggestions that are made herein are for entertainment purposes only. Professionals should be consulted as needed prior to undertaking any of the action endorsed herein. This declaration is deemed fair and valid by both the American Bar Association and the Committee of Publishers Association and is legally binding throughout the United States. Furthermore, the transmission, duplication, or reproduction of any of the following work including specific information will be considered an illegal act irrespective of if it is done electronically or in print. This extends to creating a secondary or tertiary copy of the work or a recorded copy and is only allowed with the express written consent from the Publisher. All additional rights reserved. The information in the following pages is broadly considered a truthful and accurate account of facts and as such, any inattention, use, or misuse of the information in question by the reader will render any resulting actions solely under their purview. There are no scenarios in which the publisher or the original author of this work can be in any fashion deemed liable for any hardship or damages that may befall them after undertaking information described herein. Additionally, the information in the following pages is intended only for informational purposes and should thus be thought of as universal. As befitting its nature, it is presented without assurance regarding its prolonged validity or interim quality. Trademarks that are mentioned are done without written consent and can in no way be considered an endorsement from the trademark holder.

Table of Contents

Introduction

Most women over 50 feel as if they have lost their ability to be attractive, healthy and feel good in their own bodies. This is due to the fact that in today's world, we are spending more and more time at home and we have significantly reduced our need for food. However, even if we do not need as many calories as we did in the past, most of us are still eating as if they were running a marathon a day.

Therefore, it should not come as a surprise that most women over 50 are out of shape, overweight and unhealthy. Thanks to researches and scientific studies conducted by incredible nutritionists, it is now possible to overcome the negative effect of a sedentary life. In fact, intermittent fasting seems like the perfect solution for all those women that want to burn fat, lose weight and gain a healthy and new lifestyle.

The need of all these women is what inspired the writing of this book. In fact, in the next chapters you are not going to find complicated explanations of scientific topics that, even if interesting, do not give you a clear direction on what you can do to start feeling better. On the contrary, while writing this book, a great effort was made to make sure that each concept is followed by a subsequent strategy that can be implemented in a healthy intermittent fasting protocol.

By reading this book you will get all the information and practical steps you need to follow to start intermittent fasting in just a few days. We advise you to talk to your doctor before changing your diet as intermittent fasting is not suitable if you have certain healthy conditions.

Please, be aware that the goal of this book is to give you accurate information on intermittent fasting, but it does not take the place of a professional opinion. We hope that you can find motivational and informative insights that help you make a change for the better.
To your success!

Chapter 1

An Introduction to Fasting

Before beginning our discussion about intermittent fasting, it is important to have a good understanding of what fasting actually is in a more general sense. In the next few pages we are going to lay out the basics for the rest of the book, so pay close to attention.

Although cases of prolonged fasting due to lack of food are extremely rare in our society, voluntary food deprivation is often undertaken for political, social or religious reasons. Since humans can survive absolute fasting for about 24-30 days, the body's physiological response to this deprivation can be divided into 4 phases, respectively called the post-absorption period, short fasting, medium fasting and prolonged fasting.

Let's take a look at them one by one to understand them better.

Post-absorption period

It occurs a few hours after the last food intake, as soon as the foods introduced in the last meal have been completely absorbed by the intestine. On average it lasts three or four hours, followed, under normal conditions, by an ingestion of food that breaks the temporary state of fasting.

In the post-absorption period there is a progressive accentuation of hepatic glycogenolysis ("breakdown" of glycogen into the individual glucose units that make it up), which is necessary to cope with the glycemic drop and supply extrahepatic tissues with glucose.

Short-term fasting

In the first 24 hours of food deprivation, metabolism is supported by the oxidation of triglycerides and glucose deposited in the liver in the form of glycogen. Over time, given the modest amount of hepatic glycogen stores, most of the tissues (muscle, heart, kidney, etc.) adapt to use mainly fatty acids, saving glucose. The latter will be destined above all to the brain and anaerobic tissues such as red blood cells which, in order to "survive", absolutely need glucose. In fact, they cannot use fatty acids for energy purposes. Under similar conditions, the cerebral demands for glucose amount to 4 g/hour, while those of the anaerobic tissues amount to 1.5 g/hour. Since the liver cannot obtain more than 3g of glucose per hour from glycogenolysis, it is forced to activate an "emergency" metabolic pathway, called gluconeogenesis. This process consists in the production of glucose starting from amino acids.

Fasting of medium duration

If food deprivation lasts beyond 24 hours, the action described in the adaptation phase continues with a progressive accentuation of gluconeogenesis. The amino acids necessary to satisfy this process derive from the breakdown of muscle proteins. Since there are no protein deposits in the body to be used for energy purposes, the body, in order to survive the fast, is forced to "cannibalize" its muscles. This process is accompanied by an inevitable reduction in muscle mass, with the consequent appearance of weakness and apathy.

In the early stages, gluconeogenesis is capable of producing over 100g of glucose per day, but soon enough the efficiency of this process decreases to around 75 g/day. Unlike what happens during the first phase, this quantity is no longer sufficient to ensure an adequate supply of glucose to the brain. Therefore, this organ is forced to increasingly resort to ketone bodies, three water-soluble molecules deriving from the oxidation of fats in conditions of glucose deficiency. The overproduction of ketone bodies (a process called ketosis), while prolonging the survival of the organism by a few days, causes an important increase in blood acidity.

During fasting periods of medium duration, which extends up to the twenty-fourth day of food deprivation, the recourse of other tissues to lipid oxidation increases more and more, with a general view of maximum saving of blood glucose.

Prolonged fasting and death

This phase begins when the fast lasts beyond the 24th day. The body has now exploited all the protein resources, including plasma proteins. The mix of ketosis, the lowering of the immune defenses, the dehydration and the reduced respiratory efficiency (given by the catabolism of the proteins of the diaphragm and intercostal muscles) condemns the individual to an unfortunate fate.

So should you be afraid of fasting? That's a reasonable question and if you bought this book is because you are interested in seeing what it can do to help you lose weight. Let's be clear from the start: no, fasting is a great solution to burn fat and get healthier. However, there are some important things to point out to avoid making bad mistakes that can result in health damages.

Many people resort to fasting driven by fashions, advertising or food and health beliefs that are at least questionable. Voluntary abstinence from food intake is understood, in these cases, as a moment of physical purification, aimed at eliminating toxins accumulated due to an incorrect diet.

To analyze this fact, after having broadly described the biochemical aspects, we can start from two assumptions. The first, irrefutable, is that we have plenty of food available, a high-calorie food that is often the basis of obesity; in short, we eat too much and the consequences are there for everyone to see. In fact, overeating and a sedentary lifestyle are among the very first causes of death in industrialized countries, including the US. The second point is that a moderately low-calorie diet, summarized in the Japanese saying "hara hachi bu" (get up from the table with an 80% full stomach), is one of the best strategies for living longer and healthier.

While many people should cut down on their food intake, there is no need to resort to extreme solutions such as prohibitive diets or fasting. Instead, it is enough, as our grandparents used to say, to get up from the table when you are still a little hungry and keep in mind that a little exercise never hurts.

Fasting, similar to physical activity, is a stress for the body. The difference is that, while sport leads to an improvement in organic abilities, fasting moves in the opposite direction. The lack and prolonged intake of nutrients reduces muscle mass and basal metabolism (up to 40% in extreme cases). Furthermore, the mind becomes cloudy and a global state of debilitation arises, characterized by a decrease in muscle strength and ability to concentrate. All this has nothing therapeutic or detoxifying.

Partial or attenuated fasting, on the other hand, could have positive implications, as long as it is applied rationally. After a Christmas dinner, for example, it is useful to follow a low-calorie diet rich in liquids and vegetables for two or three days. The important thing is to associate these foods with a certain amount of proteins, perhaps obtained from lean fish (which is usually easy to digest), and fats, for example by consuming a handful of dried fruit. In this way you avoid "cannibalizing your muscles" and depressing your metabolism excessively and then paying the consequences. This last point must also be clear to those who resort to fasting in extremis to lose weight before summer. In fact, a few pounds can be lost but the amount of energy associated with each unit of weight lost is very low. In other words, weight loss is mainly linked to increased diuresis and muscle catabolism induced by prolonged fasting.

As you might have noticed, even if this book is about intermittent fasting for weight loss, we are not advocating the use of fasting without pointing out the importance of doing things the proper way. In fact, the main reason we decided to write this book is to share the right information that can actually make a difference when starting out with intermittent fasting. Your health is extremely important and we would never advise you to do extreme things just to lose a few pounds.

Now that we are done with this disclaimer, we can finally focus on how you can use intermittent fasting to start losing fat.

Chapter 2

The Basics of Nutrition

We feel it is important to start every diet related book by giving an introduction to the basics of nutrition. In fact, our experience tells us that most people that want to lose weight, do not even know how their body works and what that weight consists of. By having a clear understanding of the two most important elements of nutrition, macronutrients and micronutrients, you are much more likely to conduct a diet that is both healthy and efficient.

Intermittent fasting makes no exception and our focus for the next few pages will be to give you a complete overview of these two macro elements of nutrition.

Macronutrients

Macronutrients are food ingredients that must be introduced in large quantities, as they represent the most important energy source for the body. Carbohydrates, fats (more correctly lipids) and proteins belong to this category. Some scientists include ethyl alcohol in the group of macronutrients; in reality, despite the high caloric value, this substance cannot be considered as such, as it is superfluous for metabolic purposes and devoid of any nutritional value. The attribution of the adjective "macronutrient" to water is more sensible, which however, having a zero calorific value, should simply be considered a food.

Whatever the nutritional plan undertaken, the three macronutrients must always appear in percentage and qualitatively correct quantities.

In the diet of a teetotaler, macronutrients together cover 100% of the total caloric intake and, broadly speaking, about 90% of the dry food weight. In reference to carbohydrates alone, an adult individual consumes a hundred kilos of carbs per year.

All three macronutrients provide energy to the body, but in different quantities and in different biochemical ways.

The proteins, which have a mainly plastic function, provide the organism with materials for the growth, maintenance and reconstruction of cellular structures. Their calorific value is 4Kcal per gram. Carbohydrates - which provide directly available energy - also have a calorific value of 4 Kcal per gram. Lipids, on the other hand, release their energy more slowly, but contain it in concentrations that are more than double (9 Kcal per gram); for this reason, they are particularly important during rest and fasting periods.

Now let's take a closer look at some of the most important macronutrients there are.

Vegetable proteins
Vegetable proteins are amino acid chains with specific biological functions but contained exclusively in cereals, legumes, pseudocereals, vegetables, fruit and oil seeds.

Before talking about vegetable proteins in detail, let's review some very important concepts to establish the quality of a protein source.

Important terms you should know

- Biological value. It represents the quantity of nitrogen actually absorbed and used net of urinary and faecal losses. The reference protein is that of the egg which has a VB equal to 100%

- Protein efficiency ratio (PER). It indicates weight gain in grams for each gram of protein ingested (3.1 for milk; 2.1 for soy)

- Digestibility (D). It is the ratio between ingested and absorbed nitrogen (in descending order wheat, milk and soy).

- Essential Amino Acids (AAE). The term essential indicates the body's inability to synthesize these amino acids from other amino acids through biochemical transformations. There are 20 amino acids involved in protein synthesis and among these 20, only eight are essential (leucine, isoleucine and valine (BCAA), lysine, methionine, threonine, phenylalanine, tryptophan). During the first few years, two other amino acids, arginine and histidine become essential as well.

- Chemical Index. It is found by calculating the ratio between the quantity of a given amino acid in one gram of the protein under examination and the quantity of the same amino acid in one gram of the biological reference protein (of the egg). The higher this index, the greater the percentage of essential amino acids.

Protein quality

In general, the protein quality of foods of animal origin is superior as they contain all the various essential amino acids. The lower quality of vegetable proteins is instead due to a lack of one or more essential amino acids. This amino acid is called the limiting amino acid.

Cereals, for example, are deficient in tryptophan and lysine, an essential amino acid whose deficiency can lead to a deficiency of vitamin B3 (niacin). Legumes, very rich in decent quality proteins, are instead lacking in sulfur amino acids (methionine and cysteine) important for the growth of hair and nails, and for the synthesis of glutathione, a powerful antioxidant able to protect our cells from oxidative stress (free radicals).

However, by correctly combining different vegetable proteins, even alternating ones and not necessarily in the same meal, it is possible to compensate for the lack of various limiting amino acids. In this case we speak of mutual integration (or protein complementation).

Pasta and legumes is an example of an excellent combination since the amino acids that pasta is lacking are supplied by beans and vice versa.

In any case, it should be noted that all the concepts expressed so far must be interpreted rationally.

- If it is true that vegetable proteins are deficient in some amino acids, it does not mean that these are not sufficient to cover the body's protein needs.

- If it is true that limiting amino acids prevent the optimal use of other amino acids for protein synthesis, it does not mean that in these cases the protein synthesis is heavily compromised.

- If it is true that the lack of combination of vegetable proteins can cause protein deficiencies in the long run, this is not valid in the short term. For example, if we dissociate cereals and legumes into two separate meals, the body is perfectly capable of regulating protein synthesis by implementing the limiting amino acids with those present in the endogenous reserves. If, on the other hand, only one type of vegetable protein is consumed for long periods of time (for example only cereals), the free amino acid stocks are "exhausted" and a protein deficiency inevitably occurs (negative nitrogen balance).

Therefore there are no particular contraindications in consuming mainly food of plant origin as it happens during the summer period. However, it is important that the diet includes the consumption of a wide class of foods of plant origin (dried fruit, vegetables, legumes, etc.) but also of some animal foods (eggs, milk, meats, etc.). In fact, an exclusively vegetarian diet, even if sufficient from a protein point of view, could be deficient in vitamins (B12) and minerals such as iodine, iron and calcium, and essential fatty acids.

Fats

Fats, also called lipids (from the Greek lipos = fat) are a heterogeneous group of substances that have in common a low degree of solubility in water. Instead, they are soluble in organic solvents such as benzene, ether or chloroform.

They are found mainly in foods of animal origin but are also abundantly present in the vegetable kingdom (oils).

Oils and fats are very similar chemically but, while the former are liquid at room temperature, the latter are solid.

There are more than 500 types of fats, classified according to their molecular structure into simple, compound and derivative. Let's take a closer look at their distinction.

- **Simple lipids.** They are the most abundant in our body (about 95%) and in our diet (about 98% of the lipids present in food are ingested in this form). They represent the main form of storage and use. Among the best known are waxes and triglycerides.

- **Compound lipids.** They are triglycerides combined with other chemicals such as phosphorus, nitrogen and sulfur. They represent about 10% of our body's fats. Among the best known are phospholipids, glycolipids and lipoproteins.

- **Lipids derivatives.** They derive from the transformation of simple or compound lipids. The most important is cholesterol, but we also remember vitamin D, steroid hormones, palmitic, oleic and linoleic acid.

Triglycerides derive from the union of a glycerol molecule with three fatty acids in turn formed by hydrocarbon chains ranging from a minimum of 4 to a maximum of 20 carbon atoms.

Triglycerides represent the storage form of fatty acids, a bit like glycogen and glucose. During the energy processes our body in fact breaks down the bond between glycerol and fatty acids, conveying them in two completely different metabolic pathways.

While glycerol is used to produce glucose, free fatty acids are transported into the bloodstream in association with albumin, a plasma protein that carries them to the muscles where they constitute the energy substrate for oxidative processes.

Fats are normally stored by our body as energy and are the building blocks of your belly. By following an intermittent fasting regimen you make sure to burn it away while keeping a good level of health.

Carbohydrates

Carbohydrates, also known as carbs in the fitness world (from the Greek "glucos" = sweet) are substances made up of carbon and water. They have this molecular form: (CH_2O), and are mainly contained in foods of plant origin.

On average they provide 4 kcal per gram, even if their energy value fluctuates from 3.74 kcal of glucose to 4.2 Kcal of starch. About 10% of these calories is used by the body for digestion and absorption processes.

Based on their chemical structure, carbohydrates are classified into simple and complex.

Simple carbohydrates, commonly called sugars, include monosaccharides, disaccharides and oligosaccharides. In nature there are more than 200 monosaccharides which differ in the number of carbon atoms present in their chain.

Hexoses (fructose, glucose, galactose) are the most important from a nutritional point of view. Let's take a look at the different types of carbs there are.

Monosaccharides

- Glucose is normally found in foods, both in free form and in the form of polysaccharide. It constitutes the form in which the other sugars must be transformed in order to be used by our body. Only 5% of the total amount of carbohydrates present in our body is represented by glucose circulating in the blood. Glycemic index = 100.
- Fructose is found in abundance in fruit and honey; it is absorbed in the small intestine and metabolized by the liver which transforms it into glucose. Its glycemic index is very low, equal to 23.
- Galactose in nature is not found free but it is always linked to glucose it forms lactose, the sugar of milk.

Oligosaccharides are formed by the union of two or more monosaccharides (maximum 10). They are found mainly in vegetables and in particular in legumes. The best known, since they are important from a nutritional point of view are disaccharides (sucrose, lactose and maltose).

Disaccharides

- Sucrose. Glucose + fructose; very common in nature it is present in honey, beets and sugar cane. Its glycemic index is 68 ± 5.
- Lactose. Glucose + galactose; it is the sugar of milk and the least sweet of the disaccharides. Its glycemic index is 46 ± 6.
- Maltose. Little present in our diet is found mainly in beer, cereals and sprouts. Its glycemic index is 109.

Among the oligosaccharides we mention maltodextrins.

Oligosaccharides

Maltodextrins are oligosaccharides deriving from the hydrolysis process of starches. They are used as energy supplements and can be useful in endurance sports. They provide short and medium term energy without straining the digestive system too much.

Polysaccharides are formed by the union of numerous monosaccharides (from 10 to thousands) through glycosidic bonds. Vegetable polysaccharides (starches and fibers) and polysaccharides of animal origin (glycogen) are distinguished. Polysaccharides containing a single type of sugar are called homopolysaccharides, while those containing different types of monosaccharides are called heteropolysaccharides.

Polysaccharides

- Starch is the carbohydrate reserve of vegetables. It abounds in seeds, cereals; it is also found in large quantities in peas, beans and sweet potatoes. It occurs naturally in two forms, amylose and amylopectin. The higher the amylopectin content, the more digestible the food is.

- Fibers are structural polysaccharides, the most important of which is cellulose. Our body is not able to use them for energy purposes, but their fermentation in the intestine is essential to regulate the absorption of nutrients and to protect our body from numerous diseases. They are divided into water-soluble and non-water-soluble. The former chelate by interfering with the absorption of nutrients, including cholesterol, the latter attract water, accelerating gastric emptying. The caloric contribution of fiber in the diet is zero.

- Glycogen is a polysaccharide similar to amylopectin used as a source of storage and primary energy reserve. It is stored in the liver and muscles up to a maximum of 400-500 grams. The glycogen present in animals is almost completely degraded at the time of slaughter so it is present in extremely small quantities in food.

In general, carbohydrates can be considered an easy to access source of energy. Most athletes take them before training as they give your body immediate energy to perform activities. When doing intermittent fasting, you want to avoid eating carbohydrates during the fasting periods as your goal is to empty the glycogen in your muscles to start burning fat.

Micronutrients

Vitamins and Minerals are nutrients that do not bring energy, but whose presence is essential for the correct functioning of the organism. They work at very low doses and are therefore referred to as micronutrients.

For people in general, but especially for athletes, microelements can make the difference in sports training; especially for bodybuilders, who often fail to meet their needs for the following reasons.

- Some have milk intolerance and do not eat dairy products due to the fat content.
- Many do not eat vegetables or fruit due to their sugar content or because they are not very pleasing to the palate.
- They consume minimal amounts of fat and not at every meal.
- In pre-competition diets they almost totally eliminate fats and carbohydrates.

It follows that integration is almost always indispensable for these people.

For example, for minerals it would be useful to carry out a blood test or a hair analysis to see if you have a deficiency or not. Most women over 50 tend to suffer from this type of deficiency and we advise you to consult your doctor to see if a supplement can help you out. Another option would be to take a multivitamin-mineral complex daily, you cannot go wrong with it. Some vitamins have a very short life (especially the water-soluble ones, which only last 3-4 hours) so it is better to use a prolonged release compound associated, perhaps, with essential fatty acids.

Vitamins

They are enzymatic substances and, similar to some amino acids and fatty acids, they are essential nutrients, as our body is unable to synthesize them. The vitamin requirement varies greatly from one individual to another, because the activity of certain enzymes can differ up to 50 times from case to case. Depending on their solubility we distinguish the vitamins into fat-soluble and water-soluble.

The fat-soluble vitamins are stored in the body and can give rise to overdosing phenomena. If, on the other hand, one or more of these substances, whether or not they are soluble in water, are supplied in insufficient quantities, deficiency problems arise. We will therefore talk about avitaminosis and hypovitaminosis.

Avitaminosis is the complete lack of a vitamin; while this problem is rare in countries in good economic conditions, it is a common plague in underdeveloped regions. Much more widespread than one might believe, even in industrialized populations, is hypovitaminosis, that is, the partial lack of vitamins; the causes are mainly found in the high consumption of preserved foods, as well as artificially ripened fruit and vegetables. Furthermore, vitamin deficiencies may arise due to the administration of drugs, especially antibiotics or due to increased needs during pregnancy, breastfeeding, growth, infectious diseases and intense physical activity.

As we already mentioned, most women over 50 are highly recommended to supplement their diet with a good multivitamin-mineral complex. Go to your local drug store and you will certainly find someone able to advise you on the best one for you.

Minerals

A mineral is a substance made up of the combination of a metallic and a non-metallic element. These "elements" are "simple bodies" that are not divisible. The universe is made up of 103 known chemical elements, of which 22 are indispensable for the organism; others are present in traces but are not essential. On the contrary, they can even become toxic, such as arsenium, mercury or lead, to the point of causing death.

These elements cannot be created or destroyed, but they are preserved integrally and cannot be transformed to cover a deficiency.

Hydrogen is the basic element from which all others are composed. In fact, 96% of the human body is made up of only 4 elements:

- oxygen;
- carbon;
- hydrogen;
- nitrogen

Oxygen represents 65% of body weight. The remaining 4% is composed of the other elements, of which 2.5% (of the total body weight) is given by calcium and phosphorus.

The chemical composition varies from individual to individual and depends on different aspects as we will see in a minute. For example a bodybuilder will have a higher nitrogen percentage than that of a normal individual. There can be significant differences in the content of mineral elements between various individuals, due to the following reasons.

- Age. Many metallic elements tend to accumulate over the years and it is not a surprise that women over 50 have a greater mineral concentration than younger people.

- Sex. Men and women have a different concentration of minerals in their bodies.

- Physical activity. A more active person tends to accumulate more minerals, especially if supplements are taken on a regular basis.

- Drugs. People that take drugs on a regular basis tend to accumulate more minerals. The higher concentration can be due to past events as well, especially if the drugs were strong.

- Eating habits. Minerals are generally found in high quality fruits and vegetables. If you conduct a healthy intermittent fasting lifestyle you should not have any issue concerning minerals.

- The environment. Certain regions are richer in terms of minerals present in the soil. Clearly, everything that is cultivated in these places will have greater minerals concentration as well.

The origin of the food is fundamental. In fact, if a certain element is not present in the soil it will not be present in the fruits and vegetables that are cultivated there. Furthermore, they will not be present in high concentration in the meat of the animals that feed in that place as well. In theory, in order to have all the foods we need, we would have to eat everything at every meal, but this is practically impossible.

Furthermore, for the correct assimilation of minerals the presence of vitamins is often necessary and vice versa. Many minerals to be active must be linked to other substances and the fat-soluble vitamins require the simultaneous presence of fats. Finally, excessive consumption of alcohol and dietary fiber can create intestinal malabsorption problems.

Considering that most of the water-soluble vitamins are eliminated within a few hours, the ideal would be to take a small amount of a multivitamin-mineral supplement with each meal. Once again, your local drug store will have everything you need. Go and ask for advice!

We can divide minerals into macroelements that are present in the organism in greater quantities and into oligoelements, that are present in infinitesimal quantities. Among the latter we still have some useful elements (zinc, iron, iodine, selenium, manganese, copper) and some toxic elements, such as lead, mercury, cadmium and arsenic. In any case, the toxicity of minerals essentially depends on the amount that is consumed by the body. This means they are all potentially toxic at high doses.

We hope that by reading this chapter you have understood the importance and the complexity of nutrition. It is a fascinating topic that could last for many more pages. However, our goal was to give you the basic concepts and help you realize that when it comes to intermittent fasting is not just a matter of not eating for a certain period of time. You have to know what to eat after your fasting as well, as your body will need to be fed properly after such a stressful event.

Especially if you are a woman over 50, we advise you to pay particular attention to your eating habits after fasting. They are what can make or break your ability to lose weight and, most importantly, be healthy. When in doubt, consult a professional doctor.

Chapter 3

Benefits of Intermittent Fasting

Now that we have discussed the basics of nutrition, let's begin our journey into the fascinating world of intermittent fasting by taking a look at the benefits it has.

Intermittent fasting is a weight loss system based on the cardinal principle of creating a window of fasting with a duration that affects the overall caloric balance and hormonal metabolism. In conditions of food abstinence, in addition to a total insulin calm (remember that insulin is the anabolic hormone par excellence but also responsible for adipose deposition), there is a significant increase in another hormone: IGF-1 or somatomedin (some even mention an increase in testosterone). The intermittent deprivation of food is then responsible for the secretion of GH (somatotropin), known as the "feel-good hormone". Unlike insulin, GH, while increasing hypertrophy, does not cause fat deposits, but favors the lipolysis necessary for weight loss and muscle definition.

The main dietary regimes that involve intermittent fasting are the following three.

- Fasting every other day;
- Fasting for 2 days a week;
- Daily fasting (the period of the day during which the individual eats is limited to 8-12 hours and the remaining 12-14-16 hours are dedicated to fasting).

Dietary pattern of intermittent fasting
The food pattern of intermittent fasting consists of 3 daily meals and 1 training session with a fasting window of 16 hours. This is what experts recommend to women over 50 that are starting this eating regiment.

This is a quick scheme of a typical intermittent fasting day.

- 1st meal to be consumed as soon as you get up. For this first meal, a protein and carbohydrates source with a medium-low glycemic index is advised. Please, avoid consuming high fat foods in this first meal.

- 2nd meal. This should be your breakfast. In this case, eat a complete meal high in macronutrients and micronutrients. Take your supplements during this meal.

- Training. We will have a dedicated chapter to training for women of your age, but in this case a light bodybuilding routing or high intensity training should be a good indication.

- 3rd meal. Consume this immediately after training. This is your lunch, so make sure you eat your carbs, proteins and fats.

- Fasting window from about 1:00 pm or 3:00 pm until the following morning.

Benefits of intermittent fasting

Some specialists propose to treat overweight and metabolic diseases through the so-called therapeutic fasting. This practice takes place under conditions of medical supervision and nutritional support. Fasting can be beneficial or harmful based on some factors: duration, completeness of food abstention, pathological conditions for its application, etc. Not all forms of fasting are created equal. In fact, some are extremely debilitating and harmful, others are less exhausting and more rational.

Several studies have highlighted the body's health benefits of intermittent fasting. Not only weight loss and the contrast of free radicals, which translated can seem like an elixir of life, but also resources capable of regulating blood sugar levels and inflammation. From a cardiovascular health perspective, intermittent fasting improves blood pressure levels, resting heart rate, blood triglyceride and cholesterol levels, and reduces oxidative stress related to the development of atherosclerosis.

Effects on metabolism

As we have seen in the previous chapter, the main essential nutrients for our body are sugars (especially glucose), proteins and fatty acids. After meals, excess fats are accumulated in the adipose tissue in the form of triglycerides which are broken down into glycerol and fatty acids during fasting. The liver converts fatty acids into ketone bodies, which provide energy to many organs. During intermittent fasting the levels of ketone bodies increase in the blood of humans approximately 8-12 hours after the last meal is consumed. The change in metabolism affects the regulation of glucose levels, blood pressure, heart rate and abdominal fat loss.

Effects on health and aging

Caloric restriction (i.e. the reduction of food intake) seems to increase life expectancy. In some studies, people subjected to intermittent fasting have shown the following positive results.

- weight loss;

- reduction in abdominal circumference;
- better insulin sensitivity and therefore a lower risk of developing diabetes;
- greater muscle endurance;
- increased cognitive ability.

However, there is a lack of scientific validation capable of defining whether these effects are related to intermittent fasting or to the caloric deficit alone.

The Okinawa case

The island of Okinawa (south of Japan) holds the absolute record for the number of ultra-centennial inhabitants. Here intermittent fasting is practiced regularly, mainly vegetables, seaweed, goya, tofu, fish (very raw, even large pieces such as tuna) and very little meat are eaten. Another very important aspect that characterizes the eating style of the inhabitants of this Japanese island is caloric moderation; in this regard, a famous local saying suggests eating about 80% of the food needed to feel full. We truly agree with this philosophy of life. You should never become enslaved to your food.

Long-term applicability

Despite the disparate health benefits of intermittent fasting, incorporating this practice into everyday life is not easy. In fact, during the first few weeks, most people have to deal with anger, irritability, and difficulty concentrating. Before starting intermittent fasting it is necessary to ask for the help of a nutritionist or dietician to ensure a balanced intake of macro and micro nutrients. Once again, we remind you that this book is for entertainment purposes only and we advise you to see medical help before starting any diet.

Chapter 4

Therapeutic Fasting

In the previous chapter we mentioned the possibility to use fasting to cure some pathologies. Since the goal of this book is to give you every tool and information you might need to develop a healthy lifestyle through intermittent fasting, we feel it is our duty to dedicate a chapter to this important subject. The last thing we want is to have people with severe conditions reading this book and thinking they can just fast them away.

In nature, because food is not always available, intermittent fasting is part of the survival routine and any animal organism can handle it.

For humans, fasting means refraining from consuming some or all foods, drinks or both, for a period of time that can be determined or indefinite.

Absolute fasting is defined as the failure to eat any solid or liquid food for a certain period, usually between 24 hours or more than a few days.

Imposed Fast

For evolutionary reasons, the human body (thanks to its hormonal flows) is able to adapt optimally to the absence of food. The same cannot be said for overeating, as a result of which you can get sick of the so-called diseases of well-being (obesity, dyslipidemia, type 2 diabetes mellitus, hypertension, etc.).
In this regard, some specialists propose to treat overweight and metabolic diseases through the so-called therapeutic fasting. This practice takes place under conditions of medical supervision and nutritional support (with food supplements and water taken on a regular basis).

As we have seen in previous chapters as well, fasting can be beneficial or harmful based on some factors.

For example: duration, completeness of food abstention or nutritional support, medical control, pathological conditions for its application, etc.

Fasting, whether controlled or uncontrolled, therapeutic or not, is still very stressful for the body and mind. However, its potential harmfulness mainly depends on the parameters with which it is programmed.

An example of highly questionable fasting is the so-called tube diet. This is based on a form of chronic fasting, during which the body is supported exclusively by enteral artificial nutrition (nasogastric tube).

We do not endorse these types of fasting. In fact, similar practices can have the following consequences.

- Physical debility and tendency to malnutrition and ketosis;
- Limitation of physical activities;
- Food miseducation.

On the contrary, in subjects suffering from metabolic pathologies, short periods of food interruption - such as, for example, the emphasis on the night fasting period (that during sleep, taking it from 8 to 12 or 14 hours) - does not cause side effects. and favor the remission of certain metabolic parameters (especially hyperglycemia and hypertriglyceridemia) or other disorders (fatty liver, gastroesophageal reflux, etc.). Obviously, the example just reported does not represent a real fast and this is the only form of food abstention potentially beneficial and free of side effects.

Many believe that absolute fasting can negatively affect hormonal flows, specifically by suppressing the action of the thyroid gland (the one that secretes the hormones responsible for regulating metabolism); this is only partially true. In fact, prolonged fasting undoubtedly reduces the secretion of thyroid hormones. However, in general, this reduction does not occur before 24 or 48 hours.
There is some scientific evidence showing that fasting can play an important role in people receiving

chemotherapy, but more studies are needed to define its actual efficacy and possible clinical application.

Can fasting be used to cure some conditions?
Some centers specialized in the treatment of metabolic diseases use therapeutic fasting for weight reduction and for the restoration of metabolic parameters.

Therapeutic fasting systems rarely rely on irrevocable abstinence from food, and none of these prohibit the use of water. On the contrary, the tendency is to encourage the intake of liquids and, sometimes, of certain plant foods in certain portions (especially in the case of certain particular diseases).

According to the experience of the operators who propose therapeutic fasting, the greatest difficulty consists in the initial acceptance of the therapy, not in the protocol itself. Few believe people can survive 2 or 3 weeks without eating but, on the other hand, many have spontaneously reached 30-40 days.

How does it work?
The first 24-48 hours of therapy include complete fasting with the sole intake of water.

In this phase, which is also the hardest, the body consumes most of the sugar and triglycerides present in the blood. Obviously, glucose levels are kept progressively stable by hepatic glycogen, while motor action (typified by absolute rest) is mainly supported by muscle glycogen stores.

Warning! As of now, it is already quite clear that this technique cannot be used in the case of liver impairment, type 1 diabetes or other diseases that involve significant metabolic difficulty.

The true metabolic action (or rather, that sought by therapists) occurs at the end of this first phase, that is when the glycogen reserves are reduced to the bone. At this point, the body begins to burn mainly the adipose tissue, with the production and blood flow of molecules called ketones.

Sometimes, in compromised subjects or those who take certain drugs, therapeutic fasting involves the intake of vegetable juices to reduce the state of ketoacidosis.

Therapeutic fasting is interrupted in progressive matters, starting with the intake of juices and centrifuged, then of smoothies and vegetable cut in small pieces, reaching up to the intake of cereals and legumes.

Effects

Ketones, although potentially toxic, can have positive effects on therapeutic compliance. This depends on the tolerance of the patient.

In fact, by acting in a suppressive manner against the central nervous system, ketones reduce the stimulus of hunger to a minimum.

Some even claim that ketones can cause a feeling of general well-being. However, this condition called "ketoacidosis" is not free from side effects, including: liver and kidney toxicity, tendency to dehydration, hypotension, and many other conditions you need to avoid.

Fasting and digestive rest

Those who propose therapeutic fasting affirm that this feeling of well-being is not attributable only to ketoacidosis, but also to the total rest of the gastrointestinal tract.

Indeed, the digestion of subjects suffering from obesity is always a rather demanding process. In fact, by consuming very abundant meals, not very digestible and responsible for high glycemic peaks, these people are used to living with a feeling of almost continuous psycho-physical weakness.

Fasting and cell washing

A further beneficial effect of therapeutic fasting, further emphasized by the administration of antioxidant supplements, is the so-called cell washing. Not everyone knows that the organism has various means of excretion of useless or toxic molecules; among these we find the following:

- bile
- feces
- urine
- sweat

- mucus
- lung ventilation
- hair
- nails

Therapeutic fasting makes it possible to exploit these mechanisms without simultaneously taking in other pollutants or other toxic agents, among which we remember: mercury, arsenic, lead, dioxin and food additives.

Fasting and taste buds

Another great advantage of therapeutic fasting is the restoration of the gustatory papillary function of the tongue, which occurs through a process called neuroadaptation.

This perceptual reset effect of tastes is very useful for the subsequent reorganization of the diet in the maintenance phase, which involves the exclusive use of fresh and lightly seasoned foods.

Recommendations

Therapeutic fasting violates every principle of dietetics and nutritional balance. It is a radical intervention that could find application in the replacement of bariatric surgery.

It must be remembered that ketogenic diets have a very deleterious effect on the body, starting from kidney fatigue up to the wasting of muscle tissue.

Regardless of personal or professional opinion, it is important to underline that it is objectively a technique that can only be practiced within specialized structures, where medical personnel are able to supervise the entire process and, if necessary, implement the use of drugs or specific supplements.

The nutritional supplements, on the other hand, are vitamin, saline and amino acid in nature; the overall advice for those facing therapeutic fasting is to suspend any drug treatment, except for those that cannot be discontinued. In the presence of certain pathologies (organic or psychiatric), of special physiological conditions (pregnancy, breastfeeding), old age and growth, therapeutic fasting is totally not recommended.

We would like to end this chapter by pointing out that intermittent fasting and therapeutic fasting are two totally different things. While therapeutic fasting requires medical supervision during the entire process, a healthy intermittent fasting routine can be conducted autonomously by visiting your doctor once every couple of weeks.

For women of your age we encourage you to seek professional advice before, during and after this practice.

Chapter 5

Training while Fasting

Training on an empty stomach has a number of undoubted advantages in terms of lipid oxidation, deriving from the metabolic implications of morning hypoglycemia. It is no coincidence that this training technique is now widely used to promote weight loss intended as a loss of fat mass in favor of lean.

Benefits of training while fasting

Running or cycling for 30 minutes early in the morning, after an overnight fast, is one of the most popular practices for weight loss. In fact, it is believed that aerobic activity carried out on an empty stomach allows you to burn greater quantities of superfluous fat, raising the metabolism for the rest of the day and promoting psychophysical well-being. In the morning, due to the long night fast, blood sugar and glycogen stores are generally lower than the rest of the day; given the relative lack of glucose in the blood, training in these conditions promotes a greater use of fat in terms of energy. The hormonal picture is also favorable, characterized by low insulin levels and high levels of counterinsular hormones such as adrenaline, noradrenaline, cortisol, thyroxine, glucagon, and growth hormone. All these hormones promote weight loss by directly or indirectly stimulating lipolysis. The strong adrenergic secretion (adrenaline and noradrenaline) recorded during exercise significantly raises the metabolism, which remains elevated for a certain period even after the end of the training session. The important release of endorphins induced by physical activity is instead potentially useful for promoting the sense of psychophysical well-being for the rest of the day.

Training on an empty stomach, with the intention of losing weight, could lead to excessive muscle catabolism, since in conditions of hypoglycemia the amount of energy obtained from amino acids also increases. Since consuming solid foods or a protein mix would lessen the metabolic benefits induced by fasting, to prevent excessive muscle catabolism it may be helpful to ingest a few branched chain amino tablets before training. For the same reason, in order to avoid excessive protein catabolism, it is advisable not to prolong fasting aerobics beyond 30-40 minutes. Fasting workouts should be placed in a dietary context aimed at weight loss. The ideal is to combine these aerobic sessions with weight training (obviously at different times of the day) focused on strength development. Be careful though. In fact, this does not mean that you have to train with a high number of repetitions. Rather, demanding loads in perfect short and intense style will be used. This is effective for women of your age as well, not just younger athletes.

Training on an empty stomach increases the risk of hypoglycemic attacks, especially in untrained subjects or those not used to exercising in such conditions; the onset of hypoglycaemia is signaled by symptoms such as craving for food, paleness, cold sweat, headache and dizziness, excessive irritability, tremor, agitation, difficulty concentrating and risk of fainting. At the onset of these symptoms, it is good to stop running immediately. Normally, in these cases the symptoms will then be resolved by taking small amounts of foods rich in sugars (chocolates, dextrose, sweetened soft drinks, honey, raisins), followed by a more substantial meal based on complex carbohydrates. This second meal is consumed to prevent reactive hypoglycemia from copious ingestion of simple sugars.

Taking a couple of coffees or a thermogenic supplement (based on bitter orange, synephrine, mate, guarana, cola, tea, theine or theobromine), before training is theoretically useful to enhance the lipolytic action.

Before starting the workout, it is good to drink a couple of glasses of water, especially when you do not have the opportunity to drink during the training session.
Running while fasting could also induce excessive stress from a psychic point of view, especially when too many hours of night rest are sacrificed. For this reason, this practice is generally limited to those short definition periods that precede a photo shoot, a bodybuilding competition or the arrival of summer. All

this also by virtue of the fact that it is not a miraculous strategy, given that the advantages compared to traditional training are limited. On the other hand, in front of a sprinter we notice a lean and muscular body despite his training involving a negligible consumption of fat. This makes us understand, in case the concept is not yet clear, that the ideal physical activity for weight loss cannot be separated from exercises with weights and high intensity isotonic machines. This has to be combined with traditional but often overrated aerobic workouts, independently whether they are carried out on an empty stomach or not.

Even for women of your age, we recommend combining aerobic training with strength training. In the next few chapters we are going to give you a detailed description of the different types of training you can follow in order to lose weight while intermittent fasting.

Please, note how we are putting the discussion of the different training methodologies before the actual fasting programs. That's because we believe that the only way to actually burn fat while maintaining muscle mass when you reach a certain age is to implement a consistent training program.

In this book we have decided to give you two options for aerobic training and one option for strength training. Let's see them in detail.

Chapter 6

Intermittent Fasting and Aerobic Training

Physical activity, if practiced consistently and following the correct directions, can bring significant benefits both physically and mentally. Recent studies have shown that aerobic training is even miraculous for our body and to improve our mental state.

What is aerobic training?

Aerobic training or better known by the term "cardio" is widely practiced in the gym and differs from anaerobic training in the manner, timing and intensity with which the exercises are carried out. Aerobic training is done with an intensity that allows our body to use carbohydrates and fats as fuel. When an aerobic workout takes place, the body "draws" energy from the reserves of sugars and fat deposits, thus increasing energy expenditure and promoting weight loss as well. Aerobic training does not take place for long periods of time, but for a maximum of 20-30 consecutive minutes and the intensity of sports activity has normal and well-defined rhythms, not as intense and prolonged as in anaerobic activities. In carrying out an aerobic activity, a small amount of lactic acid is produced, so as not to cause sudden changes or peaks in the heart rate and always maintaining a constant and fairly consistent rhythm. The main aerobic activities that can be practiced are the following.

- cycling;
- running;
- spinning;
- boxing;
- functional training;
- cross-country skiing.

Other team sports such as table tennis or other activities that can be practiced in the gym can also be included in the list of aerobic activities.

The benefits of aerobic training

Aerobic training is important for those who want to obtain specific benefits for the body and mind. Let's see together which are the main ones. Aerobic activity can be associated with cardiovascular training. In fact, one of the main benefits of practicing this type of activity is to improve the entire circulatory system. In particular, during aerobic training, it is possible to use a greater amount of oxygen, thus helping to improve blood circulation. The benefits for the cardio-circulatory system are not only for the heart, but there has been a significant improvement in vascular function and in blood pressure parameters.

Aerobic training also brings significant benefits to the respiratory system. In fact, many scientific studies have shown that greater tissue oxygenation is obtained after practicing aerobic sports. At the respiratory level, aerobic activity improves the elasticity and functioning of the pulmonary alveoli, reducing the presence of elements harmful to the health of the organism.

With cardio training the absorption of calcium is facilitated. In this way the bones are strengthened and the muscles become more flexible and elastic. Aerobic activity, since it brings significant benefits to bones and joints, is particularly suitable for women over 50 that want to prevent the onset of bone diseases. A recent study conducted by the University of Illinois has shown how cardio training helps improve the immune system, reducing the attack of bacteria and viruses that cause colds or flu.

The advantages of choosing a cardio workout are not only physical, but several mental benefits have been highlighted by recent studies as well. Like every physical activity, aerobic efforts also help to improve general mood: during training, the body produces oxytocin, better known as the hormone of happiness, thus promoting relaxation and lowering stress levels. Aerobic training is particularly recommended for people suffering from depression or for those suffering from generalized anxiety. Among the advantages of practicing an aerobic activity, there is also that of being able to play sports in the open air, favoring breathing and relaxation.

The main differences between aerobic and anaerobic training

When it comes to aerobic and anaerobic training, it is necessary to highlight what the main differences between these two types of physical activity are. Aerobic training mostly consists in the repetition of exercises for a prolonged period of time, performed with a fairly moderate effort, without sudden variations. Anaerobic training, on the other hand, is carried out by performing short-duration exercises for a limited period of time, but employing greater effort.

The differences between aerobic and anaerobic training do not only concern the way in which the exercises are performed, but also how the body responds to these stimuli. In fact, aerobic training draws energy from sugar and fat stores, while anaerobic training draws it from sugar reserves, muscles and liver, so that you have to stop exercising after a few minutes to allow the body to restore the energy consumed. During aerobic training there is a large production of lactic acid, while in cardio, the production of lactic acid is limited. The two types of training produce different effects on the body. In fact, those who practice aerobic activity tend to lose weight fast, while those who exercise anaerobically increase muscle mass and strengthen certain parts of the body.

This is the reason why we recommend to implement both of them for reaching a great level of wellbeing.

How aerobic training can help weight loss

Cardio training is particularly suitable for those women who want to lose weight. In fact, if combined with a balanced intermittent fasting regimen, it can help you lose excess pounds with ease.

Aerobic activity is by definition fat burning at its finest. In fact by drawing on the fat storage reserves, it accelerates metabolism and promotes weight loss, and also helps to decrease cholesterol and triglyceride levels. For example, jogging allows you to slim your body and make your legs leaner, but at the same time it tones and makes your muscles and joints more flexible. Swimming, which has always been considered a "complete" sport, allows you to lose weight and lose excess pounds and at the same time improve flexibility, endurance and muscle tone.

What to eat after aerobic training

Many people, after having performed an aerobic activity outdoors or in the gym, do not want to risk compromising their efforts by consuming too much caloric food. If you train early in the morning, you need to have a fruit-based snack before starting your workout. We recommend you a banana, mango and cocoa-based smoothie, while snacks and coffee are to be avoided.

To restore energy after an aerobic workout, it is necessary to consume mainly carbohydrates and limit the intake of proteins. In particular, for a post-workout lunch or dinner you can have legumes, wholemeal pasta and cereals, but not in excessive quantities. In combination with carbohydrates, you can consume lean chicken and turkey meat and as always fruit and vegetables are the best foods if you want to keep your vitamins high.

Now that we have discussed the basics of aerobic training, we would like to give you a little training program for two aerobic activities you can do without too much equipment. First of all, we are going to provide you with an easy to follow running program that will get you started even if you have never run a mile in your life. Secondly, we will explain how you can implement cycling with intermittent fasting. In particular, we recommend you to choose cycling over running if you have joint problems, as it is less stressful for your body.

Intermittent fasting and running

As we mentioned before, we advise you to go for your aerobic activity before eating. If you will decide to follow our basic intermittent fasting program (more on that in the next chapters), this means you will run in the morning. On the other hand, if you go with our more advanced fasting program (once again, more on that later), you will go for a run before lunch.

In both these scenarios you can follow this easy running program to start from zero and work your way up to 5km (3.1 Miles) in one running session.

	Week 1	Week 2	Week 3	Week 4	Week 5	Week 6
Monday	5 min walk, 1 min run, 1 min walk (repeat 5 times), 5 min walk	5 min walk, 1 min run, 1 min walk (repeat 5 times), 5 min walk	5 min walk, 2 min run, 1 min walk (repeat 5 times), 5 min walk	5min walk, 5min run, 1min walk (repeat 3 times), 5min walk	5 minutes of walking, 12 minutes of running, 2 minutes of walking, 6 minutes of running, 5 minutes of walking	5 minutes of walking, 16 minutes of running, 2 minutes of walking, 6 minutes of running, 5 minutes of walking
Tuesday	Rest	Rest	Rest	Rest	Rest	Rest
Wednesday	5 min walk, 1 min run, 1 min walk (repeat 5 times), 5 min walk	5 min walk, 1 min run, 1 min walk (repeat 8 times), 5 min walk	5min walk, 3min run, 1min walk (repeat 4 times), 5min walk	5 min walk, 6 min run, 1 min walk (repeat 3 times), 5 min walk	5 minutes of walking, 14 minutes of running, 3 minutes of walking, 6 minutes of running, 5 minutes of walking	5 minutes of walking, 18 minutes of running, 2 minutes of walking, 8 minutes of running, 5 minutes of walking
Thursday	Rest	Rest	Rest	Rest	Rest	Rest
Friday	5 min walk, 1 min run, 1 min	5min walk, 1min run, 1min	5min walk, 4min run, 1min	5 min walk, 7 min run, 1 min walk	5 minutes of walking, 16 minutes of running, 2	5 minutes of walking, 22

	walk (repeat 5 times), 5 min walk	walk (repeat 10 times), 5min walk	walk (repeat 3 times), 5min walk	(repeat 3 times), 5 min walk	minutes of walking, 7 minutes of running, 5 minutes of walking	minutes of running, 2 minutes of walking, 10 minutes of running, 5 minutes of walking
Saturday	Rest	Rest	Rest	Rest	Rest	Rest
Sunday	30min walk	30min walk	10 minutes of walking, 10 minutes of running	20 minutes of walking, 10 minutes of running	10 minutes of walking, 20 minutes of running	5 km (3.1 Miles)

As you can see, the total time per training session is not very long and it almost never goes over 30 minutes. We feel that this is the optimal duration for an aerobic training session for women over 50 years of age, as you want to dedicate more time to strengthen your muscles rather than losing fat. Intermittent fasting will do that for you.

Intermittent fasting and cycling

Before moving on to the anaerobic training programs, let's take a quick look at how you can start cycling. As mentioned before, this is a great physical activity for women of your age that suffer from joints related pain and prefer aerobic efforts that are less stressful for the body.

If you have never used a bicycle before, we recommend you start by following this little program that will get you in shape to go for a ride of 60 minutes. Since cycling burns less calories than running, you will need to train for a longer period of time to burn the same amount.

	Week 1	Week 1	Week 1	Week 1	Week 1	Week 1
Monday	20' ride	25' ride	30' ride	35' ride	40' ride	45' ride
Tuesday	Rest	Rest	Rest	Rest	Rest	Rest
Wednesday	20' ride	25' ride	30' ride	35' ride	40' ride	45' ride
Thursday	Rest	Rest	Rest	Rest	Rest	Rest
Friday		25' ride	30' ride	35' ride	40' ride	45' ride	30' ride
Saturday		30' ride	35' ride	40' ride	45' ride	45' ride	Rest
Sunday	Rest	Rest	Rest	Rest	Rest	60' ride

Now that we have seen how to start cycling even if you have never ridden a bicycle before, we can focus our attention on what type of strength training to perform while following an intermittent fasting regiment. The next chapter will tell you everything about it.

Chapter 7

Intermittent Fasting and Strength Training

Even though weight training in the gym is no longer an area reserved for men, muscle development and strength training for women are still scary at times. In fact, the fear of getting too muscular and losing female curves is widespread and prevents many women from practicing strength training or weight lifting. In particular, when it comes to losing a few pounds or reducing body fat, strength training is the key to success.

Many movie, music and sports stars practice it and post the results of their favorite workouts or exercises on social networks. In fact, strength training is an indispensable ally for achieving a dream silhouette and these stars know what they have to do to stay in shape.

As a woman over 50 years of age, is it possible to lose weight thanks to strength training?

Let's start from the basics. To lose weight it is essential to reach a caloric deficit. By exercising, you help the weight loss process by increasing your calorie consumption and maintaining muscle tone. If you additionally do strength exercises, you signal to your body that it still needs to keep the muscles active and in turn it counteracts muscle loss. The consequence is that you lose weight and your body is fitter and more toned.

Aerobic training is not enough

It is often noted that in the gym women mostly use cardio equipment and avoid weights and strength-training tools. But the key to success for having a toned and defined body is strength training.

Muscle mass, which is 22% of the total body mass, consumes almost a quarter of our daily energy balance. Muscles are the most powerful weapon against excess pounds and fat pads. Muscles burn calories even at rest and increase the basal metabolism which stimulates long-term fat burning.

Strength training for women not only serves to develop quality muscle mass, but also contributes to the maintenance of existing muscles. A pure resistance training combined with a low calorie diet allows you to reach the caloric deficit, but in the long term the weight loss also results in loss of muscle mass.

The loss of muscle mass lowers the body's energy needs, which often continues even after weight loss.

The consequences are the following.

- it becomes more and more difficult to reach the calorie deficit and therefore to burn fat;
- after the first few weeks, the risk of the so-called "yoyo effect" is real.

And here comes strength training that helps maintain, defines existing muscles and promotes fat burning.

Endurance training is an intelligent integration of strength training. It helps burn additional calories, improve performance and strengthen the cardiovascular system.

Don't be afraid of getting too muscular
The fear of getting too muscular by engaging in weightlifting or strength training is totally unfounded. Women are biologically programmed differently from men. They have the same muscle structure, but typically produce much less testosterone, a hormone that promotes muscle development. The woman's body also differs from the male one in terms of muscle development, strength and fat percentage. For these reasons, there is no danger of becoming a little cube of muscles, but training will help you acquire a rounded and defined shape.

To stimulate the muscles during training and achieve good definition, you need adequate resistance. Even if you are over 50, do not be afraid to go heavy in the gym. Lift with your heart and use your muscles, they want to be used!

The benefits of strength training for women

Defined and toned shapes are one of the many advantages of strength training for women. The whole body is toned and the muscles are defined, two aspects that make a woman's body more beautiful as well. By increasing the percentage of muscle mass and decreasing fat, the lines are more defined and the feminine curves stand out more.

Unlike aerobic training, in strength training you can train individual muscles or muscle groups, thus modeling certain parts of the body.

The proportions of the body can therefore be changed, creating a more harmonious silhouette. For example, a large pelvis can be balanced by training and developing the upper body. In addition, strength training also contributes to improving the general state of health and the feeling of well-being in women over 50.

Better body awareness increases quality of life and daily well-being - those who are comfortable in their body gain more self-confidence and self-awareness.

Training in particular for the back, arms and pectorals improves posture and is especially useful for preventing the negative consequences of sedentary work.

An advantage for women with little time and limited budget is that strength training can also be done at home, without necessarily having to join the gym. Using fitness equipment, such as kettlebells or dumbbells, it is possible to perform an effective workout even at home. It only takes half an hour to effectively train the whole body.

How long and how many times a week should you do strength training as a woman over 50?
The frequency of strength training depends on your starting point. For beginners, 2 training sessions per week is already enough, while if you are already experienced and well trained you can easily train the whole body 3 times a week. Make sure you give your muscles enough time to recover and plan at least one rest day between workouts. Muscle growth occurs during the recovery phase. Therefore, in this case the fundamental rule of life applies: less is more.

When training strength, you don't need to spend hours in the gym. If you want to develop muscles, your training should not last more than 60-90 minutes. If you train for too long, the stress hormone, called cortisol, is released. This can lead to a lack of results and cause you to no longer see progress.

Also, don't forget to increase the difficulty of your exercises over time. You can do this, for example, by increasing the reps or by using a heavier weight. Important: a clean execution always remains the focus of your training!

Effective exercises for a dream body
Especially the fundamental exercises, in strength training for women, are very effective for training the synergy between the different muscle groups. This aspect is essential for a correct and healthy posture and for performing movements well in daily life and in sport. It is no coincidence that these exercises have established themselves as true classics.

The most important fundamental exercises are: weight lifting, squats, lunges, Bench Press, pull-ups.

The unbeatable benefits of the fundamental exercises are the following.

- they train multiple parts of the body at the same time;
- minor muscle groups are also involved and are often neglected in other exercises;
- thanks to complexity and effort, fat burning increases;
- they stimulate the production of the growth hormone testosterone which acts on the whole body;
- hardly any tools or objects are needed, the exercises can be performed at home and made more difficult through variations.

Example training program for women
At the beginning it is enough to train 2-3 times a week. It is possible to integrate an endurance training session. The training program can be configured, for example, as follows.

Monday	Strength training A (Bench Press, Military Press, crunches)
Tuesday	Rest
Wednesday	Strength training B (weightlifting, pull-ups, rowing machine)
Thursday	Endurance session (30 minutes of cycling)
Friday	Strength training C (squats, lunges, leg press)
Saturday	Rest
Sunday	Endurance session (30 minutes of jogging)

It is important to include breaks in your training program, as this gives your body time to recover before the next session and build new muscle mass. This is particularly true if you are on an intermittent fasting regimen, where you are constantly in a caloric deficit. To understand how to perform these exercises in the correct way, we advise you to ask your local gym instructor.

Chapter 8

HIIT: A Particular Type of Training

There is a specific type of training that we recommend to all those women that are looking to combine strength and cardio into one simple routine. We are talking about HIIT and the next few pages are going to tell you everything there is to know about it.

High Intensity Interval Training consists of alternating short and very intense efforts, therefore with a large anaerobic component, with less intense recovery periods until muscle and / or metabolic exhaustion is reached.

Duration and intensity of the peaks are inversely proportional, since the effort should be maximal or sub-maximal. Although there is no precise and advisable total duration, HIIT workouts generally last less than 30 minutes, with times that can vary according to your personal level of training.

HIIT training sessions generally consist of the following phases.

- General and specific warm up
- Repetition or series of high intensity (HIT) exercises, separated by low or medium intensity executions as active recovery
- Cool down and some exercises for flexibility and mobility.

HIT should be performed at maximum intensity, while active recovery should not have an intensity greater than 50%. The number of sets/reps and the duration of each depend on the type of exercise, but can be as little as 3 reps of 20 seconds each. The specific exercises performed during times of high intensity can vary even within the same workout. Most of the research on HIIT has been done using a cycling ergometer (stationary bike), but you can use whatever cardio equipment you have at your disposal.

There is no specific formula of HIIT. Depending on your cardiovascular and muscular level, the recovery intensity can be medium or very slow; what matters are the high intensity peaks. A common formula is a 2:1 ratio of high intensity to active recovery, such as 30–40" of fast running alternating with 15-20" of jogging or walking, repeated "X" times or until exhaustion.

The entire HIIT session can last from 4 to 30 minutes, which means it is considered an excellent way to maximize your training in the event of time constraints. The use of a watch or timer is highly recommended to respect exercise, recovery times and to estimate beats per minute (bpm) - alternatively, a heart rate monitor is very useful.

Intensity VS Volume

Intensity and volume are two parameters which, together with density, constitute the workload. In fact, the formula to calculate the total load is this:

$$intensity + volume + density = TOT\ load$$

HIIT is based, as mentioned above, on HIT (high intensity training), to which it associates IT (interval training) to be able to increase its total volume.

However, it must be said that "high intensity" is a relative concept, in the sense that it can be applied to efforts of a different nature, and which use equally different metabolisms. It is in fact common to speak of high volume training and low intensity for all undemanding aerobic endurance activities: light running for an hour, cycling for 2-3 hours, brisk walking for 90 seconds and everything in between.

In this case the intensity is objectively low; what happens though, if we report the same concept on protocols that basically stimulate the metabolisms of anaerobic intensities?

In strength training, the concept does not fundamentally change; yet the metabolisms recruited are mainly anaerobic, alactacid and lactacid. Why do we make this clarification? To distinguish the various training strategies, which obviously have different purposes.

Thinking about the training of a bodybuilder, knowing that muscle mass is sought by orienting programming in different directions, we could deduce phases with different characteristics:

- Concentric "pure" strength development: for example, with a short and rapid table, in multi-frequency in the micro cycle, based on a few exercises of 5 sets x 5 rep at 90% of 1RM, low TUT (times of muscle tension), in which the recovery is almost full

- Search for hypertrophy due to depletion of energy supplies, high production of lactic acid emphasis on isometry and eccentric phases of contraction: with long sessions of 10-12 rep at 75% of the 1RM x 4 sets, with shorter, higher recovery time, many more exercises, almost always in single frequency in the micro cycle.

This last method, which objectively prolongs the training up to 75-90', against the 30-40' of the previous one, in the context of training for muscle strengthening, can be considered a high volume and lower intensity system - also it has nothing to do with the long walks we talked about above.

HIIT is designed to increase training efficiency, both in terms of physical conditioning (muscle and metabolic), and from the point of view of infra and post exercise caloric consumption - Excess Postexercise Oxygen Consumption (EPOC) or "afterburn" or debt of post exercise oxygen.

By training in HIIT it is possible to gain a better physical condition and a higher athletic ability. In this case, High Intensity Interval Training determines an improvement in glucose metabolism (sensitivity to glucose and insulin).

HIIT vs Low Intensity High Volume Training (LIHVT)

Compared to aerobic "Low Intensity High Volume Training" (LIHVT), HIIT "may" not be as effective for:

- Treatment of hyperlipidemias, in which low intensity and prolonged training seems to act more by reducing triglyceridemia and improving cholesterolemia
- Treatment of severe obesity and uncomfortable conditions or pathologies, such as severe heart disease, broncho pneumopathies (e.g. COPD) etc.
- Muscle and bone mass restoration in subjects suffering from sarcopenia, osteopenia and osteoporosis.

However, research has shown that HIIT regimens can induce - for the same caloric intake compared to LIHVT - significant reductions in body fat mass.

Other insights, however, have highlighted that HIIT requires an extremely high level of personal motivation by questioning whether the general population can safely or practically tolerate the extreme nature of the method. This is particularly true for those that have never embraced a healthy lifestyle before.

Benefits

We now list the health effects of High Intensity Interval Training.

Cardiovascular benefits of HIIT

A 2015 systematic review and meta-analysis of randomized trials found that HIIT training and LIHVT training both lead to significant improvement in cardiovascular fitness in healthy adults aged 18 to 45. However, greater improvements in VO2 max were observed in those participating in the HIIT exercise regimen.

Another analysis also found that HIIT regimens of 30 days or longer effectively improve cardiovascular fitness in teens and lead to moderate improvements in body composition.

Additionally, a separate systematic review and meta-analysis of seven small randomized trials found that HIIT (defined as four four-minute intervals at 85-95% of maximum heart rate with three-minute intervals at 60-70% of FcMax) was more effective than continuous moderate-intensity training at improving blood vessel function and blood vessel health markers.

HIIT and cardiovascular disease

A 2015 meta-analysis comparing HIIT with moderate intensity continuous training (MICT) in individuals with coronary artery disease found that HIIT leads to greater increases in VO2 max but that MICT leads to reductions in body weight and higher heart rate.

A 2014 meta-analysis found that cardiorespiratory fitness, as measured by VO2 max, of individuals with lifestyle-induced chronic cardiovascular or metabolic diseases (including hypertension, obesity, heart failure, coronary artery disease, or metabolic syndrome) who have completed a HIIT exercise program, it was nearly double that of individuals who completed a MICT exercise program.

Metabolic benefits of HIIT

HIIT significantly reduces insulin resistance compared to low intensity training or inactive conditions and leads to a modest reduction in fasting glucose levels as well as an increase in weight loss compared to those who do not undergo a physical activity intervention.

Another study found that HIIT was more effective than continuous moderate-intensity training in reducing fasting insulin levels (31% decrease and 9% decrease).

HIIT and fat oxidation

A 2007 study looked at the physiological effects of HIIT on fat oxidation in moderately active women.

Study participants performed HIIT (defined as ten sets of 4' cycling repetitions with an intensity of 90% VO2max followed by 2' rest) on alternate days, for a period of 2 weeks. The study found that 7 HIIT sessions over a 2-week period improved body fat oxidation and skeletal muscle's ability to oxidize fat in moderately active women over 50 years of age. A 2010 systematic review of HIIT summarized HIIT results on fat loss and stated that HIIT may result in modest reductions in subcutaneous fat in young, healthy individuals, but greater reductions for overweight individuals.

HIIT and brain efficiency

A 2017 study looked at the effect of HIIT on cognitive performance in a group of 318 children. The authors show that HIIT is beneficial for cognitive control and working memory capacity compared to "a mixture of board games, computer games and quizzes" and that this effect is mediated by the brain-derived neurotrophic factor (BDNF). They conclude that the study suggests a promising alternative for improving cognition, through short and powerful exercise regimens.

Application

Since the concept of "high" intensity is related to a specific athletic ability, HIIT can be contextualized in different fields. Let's take a closer look at them.

Short-lasting HIIT, with an anaerobic and lactacid base

If referred to short-duration exercises, with an alactic and lactic anaerobic base, HIIT concerns both the maximal or submaximal expression of strength / rapidity / explosiveness, and resistance to strength / rapidity / explosiveness, both as close as possible to its limit. The limiting factor is always lactic acid. For example, in the first case you could perform 3 reps of flat bench press (rep) at 90% of 1RM, interspersed with a recovery of 6-7 ", for a number of series (sets) such as to achieve the inability to continue with the workout. In the second case, however, 25 burpees could be performed in 1'00", interspersed with a recovery of 20", for a series number (set) such as to achieve the inability to continue with the workout.

HIIT of medium and long duration, with anaerobic base complemented by anaerobic lactacid metabolism

If referred to medium and long duration exercises, with aerobic base completed by anaerobic lactate metabolism, it mainly concerns the expression of resistance to speed - rapid but cyclic movement, as in running, cycling, swimming, rowing, etc. resistance to medium and long duration strength - ability used in some particular sports, such as judo and brazilian jujitsu. In these cases, for example, the ground fight requires to maintain isometric contractions even for several minutes. For instance, in the first case - as in running - you could perform 5 rhythm variations in progression of 3', until reaching 90% of the maximal pulsations, alternating them with 1'30' 'of passive recovery which should guarantee a descent of the beats up to 135-145 per minute (bpm). In the second case instead, a circuit training could be set up with various isometric stations (isometric half squat, plank, side plank, isometric dip trust, etc.) lasting 3'00" each, interspersed with 1'30" of aerobic exercise, such as skipping, running, cycling or stepping.

Types of HIIT workouts

Peter Coe Protocol

It is a type of HIIT with short recovery periods used in the 1970s by coach Peter Coe. Inspired by the principles of Woldemar Gerschler and Swedish physiologist Per-Olof Åstrand, Coe established sessions that included repetitions of 200m fast running with only 30" of recovery.

Tabata Protocol

It is a HIIT version based on a 1996 study by Professor Izumi Tabata of the University of Ritsumeikan et al. It is based on 20" of ultra intense exercise (about 70% of VO2max) followed by 10" of rest, repeated continuously for 4 minutes (8 cycles).

Gibala Protocol

A 2010 study conducted by Professor Martin Gibala and his team at McMaster University in Canada is based on a HIIT structured as follows: 3' warm-up, 60" exercise at 95% VO2max, 75" rest, repeated for 8-12 cycles. The benefits are similar to what one would expect from a steady regimen at 50–70% VO2max five times a week.

Zuniga Protocol

Jorge Zuniga, assistant professor of exercise science at Creighton University, proposes a HIIT with 30" intervals at 90% of VO2 max, followed by 30" of rest.

Vollaard protocol

Dr. Niels Vollaard of the University of Stirling proposes a 10' training routine consisting of 6-10 maximum 30" sprints.

As you can see, there are different types of HIIT training that you can do. We recommend you to follow the classical Tabata protocol as it is one of the most effective there is. If you do not feel well during the exercise, please do not hesitate to stop, drink a glass of water and rest for a few minutes. The goal is to lose weight while staying healthy, never forget this!

Chapter 9

Low Glycemic Index Foods for Maximum Weight Loss

Foods with a low glycemic index are products which, by virtue of their chemical composition and their impact on the body, cause a moderate rise in blood sugar.

Glycemia and Insulin

Glycemia, or the amount of glucose in the blood (measured in mg/dl), is the stimulating agent of pancreatic insulin secretion; the latter represents the anabolic hormone most responsible for adipose accumulation.

Foods with a low glycemic index should therefore be characterized by a low insulin index (reduced ability to stimulate insulin, with low stimulation on adipose accumulation); however, recent studies have shown that while glucose is the major insulin stimulant, it is not the only nutrient capable of doing so.

In fact, even by taking fatty acids and especially amino acids (proteins), it is possible to significantly stimulate the release of insulin.

How it works

The glycemic index is the speed with which the carbohydrates and proteins of a food are digested, absorbed, possibly transformed by the liver, and re-released into the blood in the form of glucose. In other words, the glycemic index corresponds to the speed with which the blood sugar rises after a meal (we leave other more accurate definitions to the scientific literature). This characteristic of foods varies according to some factors: chemical composition in macronutrients (carbohydrates, proteins and lipids), relative digestibility, molecular structure of carbohydrates (simple or complex, glucose, fructose or galactose), quantity of viscose fibers, presence of free amino acids and prevalence of some amino acids over others. As you may imagine, it is a pretty complicated subject.

In general, foods with a low glycemic index are characterized by the following things.

- Presence of viscous fibers in sustained doses;
- high quantities of water;
- complex carbohydrates or monosaccharides that require hepatic transformation into glucose (fructose and galactose);
- presence of lipids;
- presence of slightly denatured proteins;

All these factors contribute to reducing the glycemic index of a specific food and a complete meal.

Biases and Truths

Recently, foods with a low glycemic index are being attributed an essential importance in the success of weight loss and it seems that this characteristic is even more important than the chemical-nutritional nature of the foods in question (carbohydrates, proteins, lipids) or the portions with which they are consumed. However, we cannot agree with this point of view.

Foods with a low glycemic index are absolutely recommended and, without a doubt, have a better metabolic impact than that of medium or high glycemic index foods. However, the glycemic index of foods is directly subordinated to any association with other foods (therefore it would be more correct to speak of the glycemic index of the meal) and to the degree/type of cooking to which they are subjected. Furthermore, even considering that the presence of proteins and (above all) fats contributes to the reduction of the glycemic index itself, we remind you the following.

- Lipids are a "ready to deposit" substrate
- Dietary protein amino acids (such as carbohydrates), if in excess, are converted and stored in the form of fat.

This statement should lead readers to reflect on the fact that, on balance, the glycemic index is a characteristic that subordinates the energy density of the food itself. Furthermore, assuming that these are foods with a low glycemic index with a modest content of proteins and lipids, we remind you that even the portion of the food introduced is of fundamental importance since it determines the "glycemic load", that is the overall "quantity" of glucose poured into the circulatory system. It goes without saying that the greater the amount of glucose in the blood, the greater the pancreatic urge to produce insulin.

There are two different classifications of the food glycemic index and different translation tables. Some of them use "white bread" as a parameter of comparison, and others a "solution of glucose and water". This last one is the most recommended, since glucose should be the nutrient with the greatest insulin-stimulating power.

The only big defect of this kind of estimation is the experimental variability. In fact, every research institution that has observed the glycemic impact of foods has obtained results different from each other. The variables that could have had the greatest impact on this diversity are the following.

- level of maturation of the food;
- sample/research subjects;
- level of cooking;
- degree of hydration of the food.

Below we will report those that, uniquely, have been classified as foods with a low glycemic index (the values refer to the comparison with the glucose solution, with a value equal to 100). We urge readers to pay particular attention to food claims as, where not specified, no heat treatment "should" have been applied. On the other hand, the doubt arises that some data may have been omitted or neglected, since the administration of raw legumes and cereals would not always be easy to apply, risking the onset of some side effects affecting the intestine (due to non-digestible components). However, considering that foods with a high glycemic index reach values even higher than those of the glucose solution itself (e.g. maltodextrin or other artifact foods), we think that an increase of some points during the cooking process may be of little importance. Certainly foods with a low glycemic index, even after cooking, will never exceed the threshold of 50-55 points.

In the table on the next page you can find some examples of foods with a low glycemic index.

Low glycemic index foods	Glycemic index
Spices, shellfish (various), herbs (various)	± 5
Zucchini, avocado, tofu, ginger, soy, spinach, shallot, celery, radish, black currant, rhubarb, leek, pine nut, pistachio, peppers, pesto, olives, chilli, walnuts, hazelnut, lupine, almond, salad (various types), endive, sprouts, champignons, fennel, carob flour, grass, bran (various), onion, sauerkraut, cucumber, pickled cucumber, Brussels sprouts, cabbage, cauliflower, broccoli, chard, asparagus, peanuts, cashews, common alchechengi, agave syrup	± 15
Lemon juice (natural), soy yogurt, cooking soy, tamari sauce (natural), ratatouille or caponata, eggplant, bamboo shoots, granular fructose, heart of palm, dark chocolate (> 85%), artichoke, Antillean cherries, bitter cocoa, gooseberries or kiwis, skimmed yogurt	± 20
Pumpkin seeds, currants, whole hazelnut puree, whole almond puree, dried peas, peanut paste, pearl barley, blackberries, green lentils, raspberry, hummus, strawberries, soy flour, kidney bean, mung bean (soy), dark chocolate (70%), cherries	± 25
Soy, turnips, grapefruit, tomatoes, pears, sugar-free jam, mandarin/clementine, yellow lentils, lentils, skimmed milk, whole milk powder, oat milk, soy milk, almond milk, fruit of the passion, candied fruit, ricotta, chickpeas, carrots (raw), raw beetroot, garlic, apricots	± 30
Flavored Soy Yogurt, Tomato Juice, Mustard, Celeriac, Tomato Puree, Wild Rice, Quinoa, White Almond Puree, Plums, Sun Dried Tomatoes, Fresh Peas, Nectarines, Peaches, bread, dehydrated apples, apples, compote apples, pomegranate, apple-cinnamon, quince, corn, linseed, sesame seeds, poppy seeds, brewer's yeast, dry yeast, sunflower seeds, ice cream with fructose, fig, chickpea flour, falafel, red beans, black beans, borlotti beans, canned chickpeas, cannellini beans, azuki.	± 35

Chapter 10

Practical Steps to Get Started with Intermittent Fasting

In the previous chapters we have laid out the foundations for what is coming in the next pages. In fact, if you have gone through the previous chapters, by now you should have a clear idea on what intermittent fasting is, how it works and have some basic concepts of nutrition.

In this chapter we get on the bread and butter of this book. In fact, we will tell you how to practically start an intermittent fasting plan.

Intermittent fasting involves an overall change in diet and lifestyle, because instead of reducing calorie intake or eliminating certain food groups, it regulates the hours during which you can eat. Typically, fasting also includes hours of sleep and prohibits eating until it ends. There are several ways to implement the intermittent fasting diet. Furthermore, it is possible to combine it with physical exercise and/or the reduction of calories in order to alleviate the inflammatory processes at a systemic level, but it is also able to lose weight and increase muscle mass.

Let's see the practical steps to start an intermittent fasting program.

Consult your doctor before starting

Talk to your doctor and explain that you are considering intermittent fasting. Ask about the positives and negatives of this diet, and be sure to let him know about any health problems you may be suffering from.

Intermittent fasting can have a significant effect on your daily metabolism. Do not fast without consulting your doctor in case of pregnancy or major medical conditions.

Warning: due to the intermittent frequency of food intake, type 1 diabetics following this dietary regimen may have difficulty regulating and maintaining normal insulin levels.

Choose time frames that you can stick to

When following this diet, you fast at certain times of the day (typically 16-20 hours a day) or even for 23 hours before making a full meal for the remaining 1, 4, or 8 hours. Intermittent fasting not only allows you to lose weight, but is also a great way to regulate and plan your food intake. It is important to establish and respect the times of daily fasting. For example, you can gradually adopt this regimen by having only two meals a day. Choose a time to have your last meal of the day and stick to it.

Choose and respect the schedule

You must opt for times that allow you to take in about 2000 calories in the space of 24 hours if you are a man or 1500 if you are a woman. Rarely (or occasionally) you can indulge in snacks of 20-30 calories maximum until the end of the fasting window (a few sticks of carrot / celery or a quarter of an apple, 3 cherries, grapes / raisins, 2 small crackers or 30g of chicken / fish or something similar). In general, the times of intermittent fasting are essentially the same, they differ only by a few hours. You can choose between several methods. Some of the most popular ones are the following.

- **One meal window**. You fast for 23 hours a day and choose an interval of 1 hour a day (for example, 6:00 pm to 7:00 pm) to prepare your meals and eat healthy dishes.

- **Two meals Window.** You indulge in two healthy meals a day, one at 12pm and the other at 7pm. Then you fast for 17 hours after the second meal, sleep and don't eat breakfast until the fasting period is over.

- **Alternate days.** You fast on Mondays and Thursdays, but eat right on the other 5 days. Thus, the last meal could fall on Sunday evening, for example at 8pm. This method is called the "5: 2 diet" and allows you to eat 5 days and fast for the remaining 2 days.

Moderately decrease your daily calorie intake

If you typically consume 2000-3000 calories per day, you can reduce this amount slightly during the shorter intervals when you can eat. Try not to exceed 1500-2000 calories per day. To achieve this, customize your diet by including healthy carbohydrates, avoiding white bread and pasta, but incorporating complex carbohydrates and certain types of fats.

You will need to take in all your daily calories during one or two time windows when you are allowed to eat.

You may find that it's not that hard to cut down on calories because you won't have much time to consume them during the week.

Don't drastically change your diet

When you adopt intermittent fasting, you don't have to eliminate any particular food group (such as fat or carbohydrates). As long as you follow a healthy and balanced diet and don't exceed 2000 calories per day you can feed yourself as you always did before starting. Intermittent fasting changes the timing of food consumption, not the choice of dishes to eat.

However, if you find yourself consuming too many processed foods, we advise you to seek medical help from someone that is qualified to prescribe you a nutritional plan. Having healthy eating habits in the first place is the first step to a successful intermittent fasting diet.

A balanced diet includes only small amounts of processed foods, which are rich in sodium and added sugars. Opt for healthy proteins (from meat, including chicken and fish), fruits and vegetables, and moderate daily amounts of carbohydrates.

Gradually adopt the intermittent fasting diet

If you are not used to fasting, this regimen can affect your appetite, hunger and body functioning. You can adopt it little by little by extending the hours of fasting between meals or by starting not to eat one day a week. It will be beneficial to your body as it will allow it to detoxify and relieve unwanted symptoms (including headaches, low blood pressure, fatigue and irritability).

You can also indulge in some light snacks at first during fasting periods. A 100-calorie snack of proteins and fats (nuts, cheese, or protein bars) will not affect the effectiveness of the fast, neither at the start nor at the end. So, eat something very light.

In the meantime, gradually change your diet by reducing your consumption of processed foods, such as sausages, dairy products, and sodas.

Have the last meal before fasting

During the last meal before fasting, don't give in to the temptation to gorge yourself on junk food, sugars, and processed foods. Opt for fresh fruits and vegetables and get plenty of protein so you don't lower your energy levels. For example, you might consider chicken breast, a piece of garlic bread, and a salad made of lettuce, tomato, sliced onion, topped with vinaigrette.

Some people binge at first, although this behavior complicates digestion and impairs adaptation to the fasting phase in the period of food abstinence.

Eat a full meal before starting the fast. If you only consume foods rich in sugar or carbohydrates, you will be hungry again in a short time.

Load up on protein and fat when you can eat. It is not easy to maintain a low intake of carbohydrates and lipids because the sense of satiety is not satisfied and one always feels hungry during the fasting period.

Refrain from food when you sleep

That way you won't think about your stomach rumbling during a long fast. Get at least 8 hours of sleep each night and fast for at least a few hours before and after. When you wake up you will no longer be hungry because you know that you will soon be able to indulge in a big meal.

The first or main meal after fasting is the reward for being able to abstain from food. You'll be hungry, so indulge in a full meal.

Stay hydrated

Although you have chosen to fast during the day, this does not mean that you need to stop drinking. Indeed, it is essential to stay hydrated during your abstinence from food, so that the body continues to function properly. Opt for water, herbal teas, and non-calorie drinks.

By drinking you will also avoid feeling hunger pangs because liquids fill the stomach.

Set a goal for weight loss

The intermittent fasting diet can actually help you lose weight by decreasing your daily calorie intake and allowing your body to burn fat stores. By reducing the time you spend eating, you can shed excess body fat and speed up your metabolism. With intermittent fasting you will also be able to alleviate systemic inflammatory processes.

If you are fasting because you are motivated by the desire to achieve a personal goal, you will have more mental strength to continue when things get difficult.

Increase lean muscle mass while fasting

This diet offers you an excellent opportunity to build muscle. Work out just before your first meal (or, if you eat twice a day, do it between meals). Your body will be able to use calories more effectively, so try to consume about 60% of your daily calories immediately after training. To stay healthy and gain muscle mass, don't cut your calorie intake to less than 10 calories per 500g of body weight.

For example, a 60kg woman should consume at least 1200 calories per day to lose weight without starving, by combining this regimen with moderate training. If you eliminate an excessive amount of calories you risk getting sick and not toning the muscle structure.

Customize your workout so you have the physique you want

The sport to choose during the intermittent fasting diet depends on the results you want to achieve. If you're simply trying to lose weight, focus on aerobic activity and cardiovascular exercise (like the ones described in the dedicated chapter). If you want to gain and tone muscle mass, you will need to opt for anaerobic training, such as weight lifting. Again, refer to the previous chapters for a detailed training plan.

If you want to lose weight, do aerobic or cardiovascular exercise in long sessions.

If you want a more muscular body, opt for anaerobic activity, characterized by intense but short-term efforts, which do not suddenly accelerate the heart rate. As we have already seen, this type of training is based on resistance exercises or weight lifting, not on long sessions of aerobic or cardiovascular activities.

Chapter 11

Before Fasting

If in the previous chapter we have talked about the basic strategies to start fasting, now we have to point out some key concepts to follow in order to start your intermittent fasting diet with ease.

By following these ideas, you make sure to stay healthy and safe from the start. Once again, if you have questions, doubts or are not sure on how to approach this diet, follow the advice of your doctor.

Fasting means stopping food and drink for a specific period. People choose to fast to cleanse their digestive system, to lose weight, and in some cases, for spiritual or religious reasons.

Consult your doctor well in advance

During the fasting period, taking certain medications could be dangerous and have adverse effects on your health due to changes in blood chemistry. Fasting may not be suitable for people with particular health conditions, such as pregnancy, advanced cancer, low blood pressure, etc. Furthermore, your doctor will likely give you a urine or blood test before the fast begins.

Determine the type and duration of fasting you want to practice

Among the numerous ways of fasting we find water fasting, juice fasting, spiritual fasting, slimming fasting, etc. As we have seen, fasting can be extended from 1 to 30 days, depending on your specific goal. Research different fasting practices and choose the one that best suits your health condition and needs.

Be prepared for the changes that will take place in your body

As a result of the detoxification process, fasting can cause side effects such as diarrhea, exhaustion, fatigue, weakness, increased body odor, headache and more.

Consider taking a vacation from work or taking some time to relax throughout the day to limit the effects of fasting on your body.

It is important to know in advance the possible side effects caused by fasting, make sure that your research and your information are correct, detailed and comprehensive.

1 to 2 weeks before you start your fast, reduce your normal intake of addictive substances and break your eating habits. This procedure will reduce the potential withdrawal symptoms that you may experience during the fasting period. Addictive substances include alcohol, caffeinated beverages (such as tea, coffee, and carbonated drinks), cigarettes, and cigars.

Change your diet 1 to 2 weeks in advance
This means following these simple advice.

- Reduce your intake of chocolate and other foods that contain refined sugars and high percentages of fat.
- Reduce portion sizes during meals.

- Reduce the amount of meat and dairy you eat.
- Increase your intake of raw or cooked vegetables and fruit.
- In the days immediately before the fast begins, limit the amount of food you eat.
- Eat only raw fruits and vegetables, they will help cleanse and detox your body by preparing it for the fasting period.
- Drink only water and fresh, freshly prepared fruit and vegetable juices.

And most importantly, do not overthink what you are doing. We have stressed out how important it is to do things the right way, but we want to emphasize the fact that overthinking the process will not yield greater results. Just stay calm and collected during the entire process and you will start burning fat like crazy.

Chapter 12

After Fasting

As we have stated from the start, intermittent fasting is a type of diet that cannot be conducted for extremely long periods of time due to the fact that it is highly stressful for the body and the mind. Especially for women of your age, we recommend not to exaggerate and limit this diet to 2 week cycles.

Once you have finished a cycle, we recommend you follow these tips to get back to your normal eating habits.

When breaking an intermittent fasting cycle, it is important to act with caution to make it easier for the body to restore a normal digestive process. Since your digestive system will most likely have reduced enzyme production and affected stomach mucus, eating too much or ingesting certain foods too quickly could cause malaise, including nausea, stomach pain, or dysentery. Returning to a normal meal slowly and strategically will help you break your fast safely, without causing any disruption to your digestive system.

Set a deadline based on the length of your intermittent fasting cycle

It is important to know the time frame in which to stop it. Normally, the length of the fast will determine the length of time needed to break it. Do not neglect the initial stages of the interruption, otherwise you will ruin all the work done and you will stop feeling good.

For longer intermittent fasting cycles you will need to provide a break time of 4 days. The first two days you will have to limit yourself to a very slight reintroduction of basic foods, and then start adding more.

For shorter intermittent fasting cycles give your body 1 to 3 days of recovery. On the first day, you will only be able to take fruit juices and perhaps some broth.

Depending on your state of well-being, you will be able to take faster steps over the next two days.

For a 1 day intermittent fasting cycle, dedicate 1 or 2 days to your recovery. Your system may not have been placed under high stress, but you won't be able to immediately resume eating the wrong foods.

Plan your meals

Creating a specific meal plan, for the length of time it takes to reintroduce food into your system, will help you avoid making mistakes by consuming food you should avoid to keep weight off. An example of food planning (to break a four-day intermittent fasting cycle) would be the following.

- Day One. Two 240ml cups of fruit / vegetable juice (carrots, green leafy vegetables, banana, apple) diluted 50% with water 4 hours apart.
- Day Two. Plus diluted fruit / vegetable juice with bone broth and 110 grams of fruit (pears and watermelon) every 2 hours.
- Day Three. 240 ml of yogurt and fruit juice for breakfast, snack with 110 grams of watermelon and vegetable juice, lunch with vegetable soup and fruit juice, snack with 110 grams of apple,

for dinner leafy vegetables topped with yogurt and fruit juice.

- Day Four. Soft-boiled egg with fruit juice for breakfast, yogurt and berries as a snack, beans and vegetables for lunch, apple and dried fruit for a snack, vegetable soup and fruit juice for dinner.

On day one, focus mostly on eating high quality fruit and vegetable juices. To start breaking fast, especially after a long intermittent fasting cycle, you need to rehydrate your body. To do this, on the first day or two, you will only need to drink diluted fruit and vegetable juices.

To break the fast, drink 240ml of diluted fruit or vegetable juice. Avoid those products that contain added sugars and additives. In fact, you just got rid of it by fasting.

Integrate fruit and vegetable juice with vegetable or bone broth. Depending on your body's well-being conditions, after another 4 hours, you can start adding broth to your diet. In order not to overload your system, it is good to give the body an adequate amount of time between one food and another. Without the right temporal precautions, processing and digesting food would be difficult, even if it is a simple broth.

Start introducing raw fruit into your diet, especially for short fasts. If your intermittent fasting cycle has been prolonged for two weeks or more, it is probably advisable to stick to a juice and broth regimen for a longer period of time. In the other cases, the time has come to move on to solid fruit. Many fruits are rich in water and easily digestible, and at the same time loaded with nutrients and energy. Your system needs foods that are easy to assimilate, which reactivate the digestive system without straining it.

At the end of the first day or the beginning of the second, you can decide to start introducing small amounts of fruit.
Among the most recommended and tolerated fruits: melons, watermelons, grapes, apples and pears.

During this time, avoid acidic fruits, such as lemons and oranges, and fibrous ones, such as pineapple.

Fibrous fruits are more difficult to digest, while highly acidic ones can cause discomfort.

Include yogurt

It is a highly recommended food for breaking an intermittent fasting cycle. Yogurt will help repopulate the digestive tract with beneficial bacteria and enzymes removed by the intermittent fasting cycle. Such probiotics will facilitate the digestive process.

Introduce it during the second day, or when you start consuming fruits again. It is advisable to reintroduce the enzymes into the system as soon as possible, without overloading it.

Use only sugar-free yogurt, as sugar (in the processed variety and not the natural one contained in fruit) will negatively affect your health.

During this time, listen to your body

It will tell you if you are moving too fast. Some symptoms are normal, such as intense hunger or lightheadedness, as you haven't eaten consistently for a long time. In case of constipation, stomach cramps or vomiting (even just the relative sensation) it will be good to go back to taking only diluted juices and broth.

Also pay attention to the foods that you are reintroducing into your diet, in fact you may find that you suffer from some food allergy. Notice how foods make you feel: nauseated, numb, itchy or heavy in your mouth or tongue.

Introduce the vegetables again

Start with leafy greens, such as lettuce and spinach. Eat them raw and use yogurt to make the dressing. Keep eating fruit and drinking juices as your body regulates its digestive system.

After eating lettuce and spinach, add more vegetables. Eat them both raw and cooked. If you wish, you can make a vegetable soup.

Sprouts are also a great choice, as they contain numerous minerals and antioxidants that are easy to digest and necessary for the body.

Add some grains and beans. You will need to cook them well and eat them in addition to fruits and vegetables. Your appetite will grow as you reintroduce different foods into your diet.

Try nuts and eggs after getting used to solid foods. The simplest way to eat eggs is to cook them soft-boiled or beaten. Hard-boiled eggs are more difficult for the body to digest.

Make sure your body feels good before introducing multiple foods. If you digest vegetables and fruit without difficulty (for example cramps, nausea, etc.), you can decide to eat more complex foods to process. But if you have had episodes of malaise up until now, wait before moving on. Trust in those foods that your body has gratefully enjoyed.

Eat small portions

After you complete your juice intake within 4 hours of each other, you will want to start by eating every two hours or so. Your body will gradually adapt to food, and you will make progress towards larger meals.

In the end, the ideal daily meal plan consists of 3 meals and 2 snacks. Once you have reached this milestone, your body will return to normal and, possibly, will feel better thanks to the successful purification.

Chew well

Chewing food breaks it down making it easier to digest. Therefore eat slowly and allow your body to prepare for digestion. Aim to chew each bite at least 20 times before moving on to the next. This is a great idea even during your intermittent fasting cycle.

Understand that dysentery and frequent bowel movements are common symptoms following the regular reintroduction of solid foods after longer intermittent fasting cycles. On the first day, you will stick to watermelon juice and introduce grapes and pears into the second. Immediately after consuming only small portions of grapes and pears, you will experience episodes of dysentery, as solid foods will pass through your system.

Those who do intermittent fasting often experience these symptoms after reintroducing solid foods into their bodies on a regular basis. During the fast, the digestive system remained at rest and inactive. The intestinal enzymes have become unaccustomed to work. Suddenly, they are given solid food and have to reactivate in a very short time. Don't be surprised that they go wrong.

The solution is to stay on the track. In all likelihood, it's not the food that's the problem, it's the simple fact that you're asking your body to do something it's not ready for after an intermittent fasting cycle. Stick to mostly fruit and vegetable juices, accompanied by broths, and ingest something simple and solid only occasionally. Your body will readjust in a day or two.

Understand that flatulence and constipation are also common symptoms

If, unlike the case seen above, you will not be able to evacuate after reintroducing solid foods into your diet on a regular basis, do not be frightened. You are not a rare case, and you are not making any mistakes. Here's what you can do.

- Mix 1 teaspoon of Metamucil (or another fiber food supplement) and 1 teaspoon of aloe juice in 240 ml of water and drink the solution obtained before meals. The fiber supplement and aloe vera are both mild laxatives, which are supposed to promote a bowel movement.

- Avoid foods and drinks that cause or worsen constipation. Dried fruit, cabbage and coffee, while otherwise beneficial, could make your constipation worse in this case. Limit yourself to those fruits and vegetables that are easy to digest, such as plums, sweet potatoes, and squash.

Understand that too much variety, especially when reintroducing solid foods, can cause digestive problems. The key to effectively breaking an intermittent fasting cycle is simplicity. You can simply find a juice that suits your body and take nothing else for a day. The next day, find a simple, well-tolerated fruit and eat nothing else. Too many take it for granted that their digestive system is very resistant and punish it by giving it what they deem necessary, when in reality it is simplicity that it asks for. Choose the easy way out, your body will thank you.

During the first week, beware of oil-rich foods. Even foods that contain beneficial oils, such as nuts and avocados, can cause trouble for those stomachs that have only recently gotten used to solid foods again.

Initially prefer fruits and vegetables without a large oil content, then notice your body's reactions to foods that are rich in them when you feel ready to reintroduce them.

If you follow these tips, we are sure you will have no problems reintroducing a standard diet after an intermittent fasting cycle.

Chapter 13

What to Eat During an Intermittent Fasting Cycle

If the fasting component is important, when it comes to intermittent fasting nothing matters more than what you eat when you can actually consume your meals.

This is why we have decided to include this chapter that has the goal to give you the knowledge to craft healthy meals during your intermittent fasting cycle. As always, if in doubt, ask your doctor for nutritional advice.

Every single person has different food preferences and caloric and nutritional needs than others, but knowing the basic strategies for preparing a balanced meal can be of benefit to anyone. Balanced meals provide essential nutrients from various food groups, and can help you lose weight, improve cardiovascular function, and reduce the risks or side effects of many chronic conditions.

To make a balanced meal, half of the plate should be fruit and vegetables

You can eat fresh, frozen or canned fruit or vegetables, without adding other ingredients (such as sugar or salt).

The equivalent of a fresh fruit would be a glass of pure fruit juice or a handful of dried fruit. The equivalent of a serving of raw or cooked vegetables would be a glass of vegetable juice. Choose vegetables and fruits of various types: dark leafy vegetables, red and orange fruits, legumes (such as beans and peas), starchy vegetables and so on.

Eat whole grains, which should make up about a quarter of a balanced meal

At least half of the grains should be whole grain (not refined). Grains include food made from wheat, rice, oats, cornmeal, barley, and so on.

For example, bread, pasta, oatmeal, breakfast cereals, tortillas and semolina belong to the cereal group. Whole grains contain all the components of the grain. Examples include wholemeal flour, brown rice, oats, wholemeal corn flour and bulgur. Read the labels of the foods you want to buy to make sure they are whole and prefer them to refined products, such as white bread, white rice and so on.

Aim to eat a minimum of 85-120 grams of grains per day, remembering that the recommended amount for women over 50 is 170-230 grams. For example, you can eat 30 grams of pasta, rice or oatmeal, 1 slice of bread, and 1 cup of whole grain breakfast cereal.

Vary your protein sources to get more nutrients

Protein should make up about a quarter of the plate to make a balanced meal.

Eat both animal and plant proteins. The former include meat, poultry, fish and eggs, the latter legumes, nuts, seeds and soy. Choose several at each meal to get a good variety.

Aim for 140-170 grams of protein foods per day if you are a woman over 50 years of age. For example, you could eat 30 grams of lean meat, poultry or fish, 50 grams of cooked legumes or tofu.

Remember that proteins such as those contained in fish, nuts and seeds are also good sources of oils, equally essential for a balanced meal.

Add skim dairy products to get calcium and other nutrients found in cow's milk

Prefer the low-fat versions of these foods. Consume about 3 servings of dairy products per day. One serving is equivalent to a cup of milk (including soy) or a jar of yogurt. Eat 40g of plain cheese or 60g of processed cheese. Dairy products generally incorporate all foods derived from cow's milk. However, foods such as butter and cream cheese are usually not included in this group for nutritional reasons, as they are low in calcium.

If your intermittent fasting cycle ends with the breakfast, eat a full meal

To get your metabolism going, prepare your first meal of the day with foods from various food groups. Eat milk and cereals (you can choose the classic breakfast ones or make a soup), pieces of fresh and dried fruit or seeds. It is an easy to make and complete breakfast, in fact it has cereals, milk, fruit and proteins. Avoid sugary grains and fruits.

If you want a hot breakfast, make an omelet with 2 eggs or ½ cup of an egg substitute, 100 grams of vegetables (such as broccoli, peppers, and diced onions), and 30 grams of low-fat cheese.

Plan ahead for your meals

Once a week, buy all the ingredients you need for healthy cooking. Prepare several portions to eat throughout the week, or eat leftovers from dinner the next day for your next scheduled meal to save time but still have a proper intermittent fasting diet.

If you want to have a quick meal after you have finished your intermittent fasting cycle, make a sandwich with 2 slices of wholemeal bread, lettuce, onion, tomato, a slice of light cheese and a few slices of a cured meat of your choice. As a side dish, eat a salad with 2 tablespoons of dressing and a glass of pure fruit juice.

For a simple and balanced full meal, boil 150 grams of carrots, steam 180 grams of green beans, prepare 190 grams of brown rice and grill a pork chop. To drink, prefer water.

When planning meals and grocery shopping, cut back or eliminate prepackaged or pre-cooked foods, sodas, savory snacks, and desserts. If there are healthy and natural foods in the pantry, it is easier to eat well, without the temptation of ready-made industrial products.

Calculate your calorie needs

Determine how many calories to eat and how much to eat based on variables such as your age, weight and type of physical activity. Customize your meals accordingly. On many online websites it is possible to make specific calculations regarding your calorie needs. Your calorie needs or ideal portions can change substantially or undergo changes due to various variables, such as the phase of the intermittent fasting program you find yourself in that moment.

Each meal should be balanced by calculating the right proportions of foods belonging to the various food groups. For example, don't eat large amounts of protein just to get more calories, or don't completely exclude a food group to reduce calorie intake.

Always consult a doctor

Make regular visits and consider any acute or chronic medical conditions you suffer from. Figure out which foods you should eat or avoid in your specific situation. Your condition may require you to change the portions of a typical balanced meal.

For example, people with diabetes may be advised to prefer whole grains to refined ones and to reduce their consumption of fruit or juice. Those with high cholesterol or heart disease should reduce their consumption of animal products and fatty foods. Those who need to lose weight can eat more vegetables and decrease the use of butter, oil, fat, sugar or salt in cooking. Do not change your diet on the basis of general knowledge and clichés regarding the pathology you suffer from. To be sure that a modification is correct, you should always consult a doctor.

Make substitutions if you have an allergy or other dietary restrictions

If you have allergic reactions to certain types of foods, consider allergens. It may also be necessary to eliminate or substitute foods due to other health problems.

If you are lactose intolerant, include dairy products that are lactose-free or that contain a small amount of lactose, or replace cow's milk with a plant-based one, such as almond, soy, coconut, rice, and so on. Look for calcium-fortified foods and drinks or foods that are naturally high in calcium, such as sardines, tofu, tempeh, kale, and other leafy vegetables.

If you are a vegetarian or can consume products of animal origin in a limited way, prefer vegetable proteins such as legumes, nuts, seeds and soy in order not to have deficiencies.

While eliminating or limiting certain allergens, try to keep a balanced diet. Consult a dietician to explain how to meet your nutritional needs despite the restrictions and how to adapt your eating needs to an intermittent fasting regimen.

Chapter 14

Intermittent Fasting and the Right Mindset

When starting an intermittent fasting cycle your mindset can make or break your ability to lose weight and burn fat.

In fact, it is your mind that will help you keep going when things will get difficult and uncomfortable. After all, if you decide to follow an intermittent fasting cycle you need to be prepared for things to get pretty wild when during the long fasting periods. By following these tips you make sure to have a strong mind that will support you in this transformative process.

The idea of starting a diet can be daunting, especially if you are not mentally prepared for such a change.

When the mind is calm and prepared, sticking to a healthy eating plan is much easier. With the right preparation you will be able to effectively reach your goals and it will be less difficult not to fall into temptation along the way.

Be aware of recurring negative thoughts related to food

Often our diets fail because of our beliefs about food and eating. Try to become aware of your eating beliefs and make an effort to change your mindset.

We often think that on special occasions it is right to let yourself go a little. There's nothing wrong with eating a little more from time to time, but be honest with yourself about what you consider special occasions. When events like eating out, business lunches, office parties and other small events all become excuses for binging and breaking your intermittent fasting cycle, diet failure is just around the corner. So try to re-evaluate what can be considered a special occurrence.

Do you use food as a reward? Many think that after a long busy day it is normal to deserve to go out for dinner or eat a whole box of donuts. Look for alternative ways to reward yourself that don't include food. For example, pamper yourself with a long hot bath, buy yourself a new dress or go to the movies. There are many ways to reward yourself without resorting to food. Breaking your intermittent fasting routine should not be seen as a reward.

Dissociate food from certain activities

Food is closely linked to numerous daily rituals. Giving up sugar and fat may not be easy when we emotionally associate them with certain habits. Make a conscious effort to break through these dangerous associations.

Try to be aware of times when you overeat or make poor food choices, both in terms of food and what you drink. Do you indulge in Coke and popcorn every time you go to the cinema? Can't you say no to a few glasses of wine on evenings away from home? Can't you imagine a Saturday morning without coffee and donuts? If so, try to tear these associations apart.

You can do this by looking for alternatives. Do not think of food as a special treat, but consider it for what it truly is. It is just food. By making this powerful switch, you will see some immediate benefits, trust us on this.

Try changing associations by replacing unhealthy foods with healthier ones

For example, when spending the night out, play a board game instead of focusing on drinking. On Saturday mornings, when your intermittent fasting regimen allows you to eat, have breakfast with coffee, yoghurt and fresh fruit. If at the end of the day you tend to try to relax by eating, replace food with a good book or some music.

Start thinking about eating badly in terms of a habit rather than calories

In the long run, you will be more likely to stick to your diet by making a commitment to change negative behaviors rather than simply keeping calories in check. Try to be aware of when you eat bad foods and why you do it. Even if it's just half a cookie, ask yourself if you're indulging in it because you feel you've had a rough day. Do you tend to eat because you are hungry or because you feel bored? If you do this out of boredom, try to get rid of this bad habit.

Even if you don't overdo the calories, always try to use common sense. Don't eat the wrong foods for the wrong reasons.

Ask for help and support

Changing is not easy and sometimes we are unable to do it alone. Ask for help from friends and family. Let them know that you are trying to lose weight with intermittent fasting and ask them to support you. Make sure they know they don't have to invite you to parties where cheap food and alcohol will be served. Also, ask to be able to let off steam with them at times when you feel particularly frustrated or tempted. Share your goals with all the people who live under your roof. Please keep tempting foods out of your sight, especially during fasting hours.

Set goals that are realistic

Many women tend to sabotage their diet by setting expectations too high. If you want to be able to stick to your plans, set achievable goals.

Remember that a balanced intermittent fasting diet allows you to lose about 1/2 to 1 pound per week, not more. If you intend to lose weight faster than this, be prepared to fail.

You should set cautious goals initially, so you will be more likely to achieve them and have the motivation to continue.

Keep a diary

If you want your intermittent fasting regimen to be successful you cannot avoid being accountable. Go out and buy a diary to accompany you along the entire journey. Record everything you eat daily and keep track of calories. A tangible account will force you to notice your bad habits and motivate you to develop new ones.

Plan your meals

Planning meals and snacks in advance will help you avoid giving in to temptation when fasting becomes difficult. In the days leading up to the intermittent fasting cycle, make a list of the healthy recipes you plan to make. Try to get ahead, for example by buying or cutting the necessary ingredients. If you want, you can also cook soups and vegetables to keep in the refrigerator, they will be very useful for the first week's meals.

Focus on concrete behaviors

If you limit yourself to analyzing your habits in abstract terms, it will not be easy to develop greater willpower. Reviewing your concrete actions will help you kickstart the transformation.

Make a list of the bad habits you intend to change. Start with small, gradual changes. Try to commit to abandoning an old behavior for a week, then continue slowly making new changes until you reach a positive and healthy lifestyle.

For example, decide that after work, instead of watching a show, you will walk for 40 minutes. Make a commitment to stick to your purpose for a week. Over the next few days, you can gradually increase the duration of the exercise, for example by increasing the distance or the duration of your walks.

Be trustworthy to yourself

On occasions when willpower is still not enough, work to get yourself back on track, even if it can mean having to be particularly hard on yourself. Doing so will help you understand that you are the only one who has the power to change your behaviors.

Acknowledge and respect your failures. Record them in your food diary. Take responsibility for failing.

Describe the reasons that led to your failure by highlighting your disappointment. For example, write something like "I ate dessert for dinner because I chose it and feel guilty after I did it". While these may seem harsh words, many find it helpful to make it clear that they have failed. You will feel motivated to make greater efforts to be able to change in the future. Trust us, this seems a hard method but it truly works incredibly well.

Consider giving in to temptation once a week

For some women, indulging in an "out of the box" weekly meal can be a great help in staying on track. A deprivation protracted for too long could shatter the entire intermittent fasting cycle. Sticking to a strict diet may seem more feasible when you know that at the end of the tunnel you can indulge in the coveted food. If you think it might help to control yourself, consider scheduling a reward meal at the end of the week or the fasting cycle.

While at the beginning you might think that you are strong enough not to need these tricks, we highly suggest to implement them from the beginning of your intermittent fasting regimen. This way, when things will get harder, because they will, you will already have the infrastructure and the right habits set up to help you deal with the difficulties of the moment.

Be gentle to yourself and respect your mind like you respect your body.

Chapter 15

An Extreme Type of Fasting

In this chapter we would like to give you a quick overview of an extreme type of fasting that some women decide to use when they decide to lose weight. We do not know why, but there is this belief that it is possible to lose incredible amounts of fat by following what is known as water fasting.

While it is true that the numbers on the scale will go down rather quickly, it is also true that your health could be compromised if you decide to go down this path. While we advise you to avoid this extreme "diet", we know that some of you are interested in the topic. Therefore, we have decided to dedicate a chapter of this book to the best practices to do water fasting in a somewhat safe way. Again, please do not do this.

If you truly want to give water fasting a shot, consult a doctor before starting the practice.

There is no more detoxifying diet or a more demanding type of fasting than consuming water alone. It has no cost and can be used to lose weight, focus on the inner spiritual life and also to help the body excrete toxins. Short-term calorie restriction can help you live longer and healthier (if done correctly), but keep in mind that fasting can also be dangerous. Whatever your goal is, do it safely: take your time, work with a competent doctor, recognize the signs that you need to stop, and gradually return to normal eating.

Absolutely avoid fasting if you suffer from certain diseases
Some diseases can be aggravated with a restrictive diet and could lead to serious health consequences. Do not do a water fast if you have any of the following issues

or health conditions, unless clearly approved by your doctor:

- Any eating disorder, such as anorexia or bulimia;
- Low blood sugar (hypoglycemia) or diabetes;
- Lack of enzymes;
- Kidney or liver disease in advanced stages;
- Alcoholism;
- Thyroid dysfunction;
- AIDS, tuberculosis or infectious diseases;
- Cancer in the advanced stage;
- Lupus;
- Vascular disease or poor circulation;
- Heart disease, including heart failure, arrhythmia (especially atrial fibrillation), previous heart attacks, valve problems, or cardiomyopathy;
- Alzheimer's disease or organic brain syndrome;
- Post-transplant complications;
- Paralysis;
- Pregnancy or breastfeeding;
- Pharmacological therapy that you cannot interrupt.

Decide how long you want to fast

Consider starting with just one day off from food and in any case not exceed three days if you are following the water fast alone, without the support of a doctor. Evidence has shown that a detox of as little as 1-3 days can offer health benefits; if you intend to go for multiple days, however, make sure you are supported and guided by a doctor, such as in the case of fasting retreats

It is arguably safer and offers greater health benefits to have periodic but short fasts, rather than just one for more than three days. Consider fasting on water for one day per week at the most.

Proceed when you are not very stressed

Schedule this detox when you are not under stress and when fasting does not interfere with normal daily activities; if possible, you shouldn't do this when you work. In fact, you should schedule it when you have time to rest physically and psychologically.

Prepare yourself mentally

The idea of fasting for several days may scare you; talk to your doctor, read books on the subject written by people with authority on this field and compare yourself with other individuals who have water fasted before. Live the experience as an adventure, but with cautious and respect for yourself.

Gradually progress towards fasting

You don't have to start suddenly and drastically, but slowly and progressively. First of all, start eliminating sugars, industrially processed foods, and caffeine from your diet for at least 2 to 3 days prior to this detox and eat mostly fruit and vegetables. Also consider reducing your meal portions for a few weeks before your fasting date. This can help prepare the body for what it is about to experience and mentally facilitate the transition to water fasting. Consider doing intermittent fasting to eventually end up consuming only water. Such a plan could last a month and follow this schedule.

- Week 1: don't eat breakfast;
- Week 2: skip both breakfast and lunch;
- Week 3: continue as in week 2 and reduce the portions of the dinner;
- Week 4: Water fasting begins.

Drink 9-13 glasses of water for a day

Generally speaking, women over 50 years of age should drink 13 8-ounce glasses of water or other liquids (about 3 liters or so) per day. You can stick to the dose during the water fast. Make sure it's good quality water or drink filtered water at the very least.

Don't drink it all at once. Distribute your consumption throughout the day; prepare three bottles of one liter each day, in order to monitor their intake.

Do not exceed the recommended amount, as this could upset the balance of electrolytes and salts in the body, causing potential health problems.

Fight off hunger

If you complain of hunger attacks, overcome them by drinking a glass or two of water, then lie down and rest, the need for food usually goes away quickly; also try to distract yourself by reading or meditating.

Break the fast slowly and gradually

To break it up, start drinking an orange or lemon juice and then gradually add some solid food; for beginners, eat small amounts every two hours or so. Start with the foods that are easier to digest and continue gradually with the more demanding ones; depending on the length of your fast, you can spread this process over a day or more. Here is the order in which foods should be reintroduced in your diet after a water fast.

- Fruit juice;
- Vegetable juice;
- Raw fruit and green leafy vegetables;
- Yogurt;
- Vegetable soup and cooked vegetables;
- Cooked cereals and beans;
- Milk, dairy products and eggs,
- Meat, fish and poultry;
- Processed foods

Stick to a healthy diet after the water fast is complete

Fasting isn't very helpful if you go back to a high-fat, high-sugar diet. Plan a diet that includes lots of fruits, vegetables, whole grains and few unhealthy fats and refined sugars; exercise for half an hour a day, five days a week. Lead a healthy lifestyle to improve health, well-being and let water fasting be only a small part of this regimen.

Talk to your doctor before starting this process

If you are considering doing water fast, you must first consult a doctor. While it may offer health benefits for many people, others need to avoid it; so be sure to speak to an expert about your health condition and any treatments you are already taking to determine if it is safe for you to abstain from food. Your doctor is likely to decide to have a physical and blood test done before the start of the water fast.

If you are taking any medications, you should ask if you can continue taking them while fasting or if you need to change your dosage.

Fast under the supervision of an experienced practitioner

It is best to proceed under medical supervision, especially if you want to fast for more than three days or if you have any medical condition. Find a competent doctor in the field and let him guide you so that he can monitor your health during the process. Ask your family doctor if he can help you with this or if he recommends a qualified dietician or nutritionist who can follow you during the process.

Avoid vertigo

After two or three days of water fasting you may feel lightheaded when you get up too quickly; to prevent this from happening, try slowly standing up and breathing deeply before standing up. If you feel dizzy, sit or lie down immediately until you feel better; you can also try to put your head between the knees when you sit to feel more stable.

If the dizziness is severe enough to make you pass out, break your fast and go to the doctor immediately.

Distinguish normal from abnormal side effects

It is not uncommon to feel slightly dizzy, fainted, nauseated, or experience occasional arrhythmias when abstaining from food. However, you should stop practicing water fasting and seek medical help if you pass out, feel confused, have heart palpitations more than one time in a day or two, experience severe abdominal discomfort, headache or any other worrying symptom.

Get plenty of rest

You may find that you have less stamina and energy while water fasting; physical, emotional, sensory and psychological rest are an integral part of the process.

If you feel the need for a nap, go to bed; read something that lifts your mood, listen to your body and don't ask too much of it.

If you feel tired and dizzy, don't drive a vehicle and call your doctor.

Don't exercise intensely during this time

The energy level fluctuates from very low to very high, but even at the best of times you must avoid fatigue. Instead, try to follow some gentle and regenerating yoga sessions; it is a relaxing practice that stretches the muscles and allows you to do some light exercise.

Yoga and gentle stretching create well-being for some women, but may prove too vigorous for others; listen to your body and just do what you feel like. If your body asks for absolute rest, do not be afraid to give it to it.

Chapter 16

One Meal a Day (OMAD)

In this chapter we are going to discuss a particular type of intermittent fasting regimen. It is called the OMAD diet and the next few pages are going to tell you everything there is to know about it.

We are saturated with a culture of overeating and binge eating, and more and more people are exploring the concept that less can be more on many different levels. As can also be understood from the growing interest in a minimalist lifestyle, there is no doubt that we are trying to simplify our lives. So why not simplify our diet and eat once a day with the OMAD diet?

Similarly, several intermittent fasting (IF) and time-restricted feeding (TRF) protocols are on the wave of the trend. As we have seen, women are exploring different time windows in which they abstain from food or fast to improve health. Even though it is currently experiencing its best time in pop culture, fasting is nothing new. Fasting has been used throughout human history for spiritual and health reasons. From an ancestral perspective, always eating three or more times a day is not what humans have done for most of their existence, as they did not have constant access to the same quantities of food and were faced with regular periods of famine. Fasting is part of our DNA.

There are many ways to do intermittent fasting, from the simple 8-6 plan (eat between 8am and 6pm) to the fast-mimicking diet. The latter includes five days in which food can be ingested for the whole day and two with a maximum of 700 kcalories. A special way of doing intermittent fasting is the OMAD diet. OMAD sounds very exotic, but it literally means "One Meal a Day". An OMAD plan includes a fast of 23 hours a day and a 1 hour feeding window in which to eat. Normally this means waiting to eat until dinner, but in theory you can set a meal for one hour at any time of the day. Women over 50 usually practice OMAD to improve their health and energy, to lose weight, or both.

So is OMAD worth trying? Let's take a look at the things to consider.

The benefits of the OMAD diet

Given that OMAD is a more advanced type of intermittent fasting, there is a greater chance of achieving all the benefits that research has confirmed, such as:

- Higher levels of growth hormone, useful for increasing muscle and reducing fat;
- Lower levels of inflammation;
- Lower risk of diseases;
- Increased autophagy (cell recycling and repair).

Another key factor of intermittent fasting techniques such as OMAD is that natural ketosis is increased, which has benefits in terms of fat reduction and anti-inflammatory drugs. Since OMAD is longer fast, it tends to maximize these beneficial effects. Longer fasting windows give the body more time to push the benefits of fasting to the limit, while breaking the fast earlier tends to slow down these mechanisms.

Simplicity and convenience

OMAD fans love the fact that there is very little to plan with this fast (because there is only one meal to prepare!). The only plan that OMAD involves is that of the meal in which the fast is broken, to ensure that it has enough nutrients for the day.

Lower risk of diabetes

Given the characteristics of the OMAD diet, insulin levels will peak only once a day and for a short period of time (usually an hour), which means that the endocrine system is relaxed. This is in theory what connects intermittent fasting with both an improvement in cardiovascular capacity and with other diseases such as Type II diabetes or autoimmune diseases. This also leads to a lower risk of diabetes-related symptoms and other disorders directly related to diet and body metabolism.

It slows down aging

All types of intermittent fasting, but especially the OMAD diet, activate autophagy, with which the body cleanses itself of damaged cells, toxins, and waste. Autophagy also occurs in the neurons of the brain, which is why intermittent fasting has been shown to be beneficial in slowing down aging and in disorders such as Alzheimer's and Parkinson's.

Reduced calories

The OMAD diet can also make weight management easier given the natural calorie restriction. In fact, it becomes difficult to eat all the calories that you used to consume in a day in a single meal, but at the same time you still feel satisfied because that single meal is still satisfying in terms of taste, as you can cook almost whatever dish you like the most.

Chapter 17

How to Eat Just One Meal a Day

In the previous chapter we have seen a specific type of intermittent fasting protocol that can help you maximize your weight loss chances. Some of you might be wondering how to actually apply this regimen in an effective and safe way.

In the next few pages, we are going to give you practical tips to fast for one full day, which is the skill you have to acquire in order to be successful with this "one meal a day" concept.

As we have seen, fasting means voluntarily avoiding eating for a given period of time. Some people fast to lose weight, others for religious or spiritual reasons. Whatever your reason for doing it, it is important to have a very strong motivation, because fasting is going against the natural instinct to eat. Having a clear purpose is essential to be able to achieve the goal. Before starting the fast, you should drink plenty of water, eat fruits and vegetables, and ensure your body a good night's sleep. By treating the body properly before, after and during the fast, you will be able to achieve greater mental clarity and burn more fat.

Ask yourself what you wish to learn from this experience - the answers will help you decide what the purpose of your fast day is. In all likelihood, you will achieve better results if you feel motivated to maintain self-control. You may want to fast for spiritual reasons, to achieve a state of mental clarity, or more simply to obtain physical benefits. If you are reading this book, we assume you are doing it because it is a great way to get in shape while being healthy.

Ask yourself questions and reflect on what motivates you and your goals. This is a simple trick that can help you a lot, especially when things get difficult. Besides losing weight, here are a couple of reason why you might be interesting in fasting for one full day.

- Fast to detoxify your body. Avoiding eating for a day will help your body more effectively excrete toxins, mucus, intestinal blockages, and other contaminants that damage your body.

- Fast to increase focus. Maybe you need to find a solution to a problem, understand a situation better, or get your intuitive and creative mind in motion. Fasting can help you achieve a greater state of mental clarity, which will allow you to analyze your problems more effectively.

Combine fasting with meditation, yoga or sensory deprivation practice to explore the depths of your mind. Use discipline and focus to escape the stimuli of hunger.

Often, when fasting for religious reasons, it is necessary to refrain from eating only until sunset. If you intend to follow the Islamic fasting rite, for example, you will have to stop eating twenty minutes before sunrise and can start again only twenty minutes after sunset. Fasting for 24 hours has become a very popular practice among those women who want to keep their body healthy and vigorous, especially among women who practice yoga on a daily basis.

It is best not to fast solely to lose weight. Even if this is an intermittent fasting book that teaches how this protocol can help you lose weight, we suggest you fast not just to lose a few pounds. There is more to that, as you might understand by now.

Fasting promotes the body's expulsion of toxins and can help you digest food more effectively, especially if practiced regularly. However, it is by no means certain that fasting will allow you to lose weight. Refraining from eating for a whole day and then bingeing on a large meal rich in carbohydrates means, for example, forcing the metabolism to reactivate in an extremely slow way. As a result, you will not burn more fat than you would have burned by eating normally.

If your only goal is to lose weight, try eating a breakfast that contains only very few calories instead of fasting for a full day. This light meal will activate the metabolism by causing the body to use up its fat reserves.

Consider fasting on juice only one day a week

With a liquid diet you can guarantee your body enough nutrients not to force it to use the sugar reserves stored in the liver and muscles. This way you will be able to detoxify the body without risking compromising muscle tissues.

Fasting allows you to start the body's self-healing process, with the advantage of improving your general health thanks to the break granted to the digestive system. Your organs will have time to take care of themselves. Fasting regularly helps you digest food more effectively, promotes greater mental clarity, increases physical and intellectual vigor, allows you to expel more toxins, improves vision and gives an intense feeling of general well-being.

Get ready for your full day of fasting

The day has almost arrived and your first 24 hours of fasting are right around the corner. It is important to get ready in the best possible way, in order to have a positive experience.

Here are a few practical tips you can follow to maximize your chance of having a smooth day.

The day before fasting, drink at least two liters of water

Water helps balance body fluids that promote blood circulation, saliva production, body temperature maintenance and digestion, as well as the absorption and distribution of nutrients. Be careful, this does not mean that you should drink an exaggerated amount of water immediately before starting the fast. In fact, the only result you would get would be to excrete it in the form of copious urine a few hours later. The right thing to do is to start drinking more in the 72 hours leading up to the fast.

Fruit juices, herbal teas, milk, energy drinks, and any other hydrating drink are helpful in preparing you to fast. Also try to eat foods rich in water, especially fruits and vegetables.

The day before your fast, eat healthy and nutritious foods

Absolutely avoid bingeing before you fast. It is much better to reduce portions than to increase them. If possible, eat mostly fruit and vegetables to balance your body. Eating food rich in water and nutrients can help your body prepare for fasting. Try to avoid baked foods, especially those that contain large amounts of salt or sugar.

During the 24 hours leading to the fast, it is also good to avoid all packaged foods notoriously rich in sugar. The human body is unable to function properly if it is fed mainly on sugars. Additionally, processed foods tend to stay in the digestive system longer, hindering the detoxification process that should come with fasting.

If you are diabetic, ask your doctor for advice on whether you can eat a lot of fruit without compromising your health.

Get a good night's sleep before you start fasting

The next day, the body will not be able to count on the caloric intake it is used to and will not be able to fight fatigue by eating foods that provide a lot of energy. By giving your body the necessary rest, you will help it function better during the day and you can benefit more from fasting.

We advise you to go to sleep an hour before you normally do. Our experience says that that extra hour will help you a lot in your mission.

The day of the fast

If you follow the tips we just gave you, you should have no problems during the fast. However, some women might find fasting a bit more challenging than others and need a bit more help to go through the process. The next few pages are full of interesting tricks you can apply to maximize your chances of success.

Please, always be aware that there is a difference between feeling challenged by the fast and feeling sick. If you do not feel well during the practice, just break the fast and eat something sweet to boost your sugar levels. If that does not help you feel better, call your doctor and ask for medical advice. Always have respect for yourself and your body.

Focus on the purpose of your fast

Direct your attention to the topics or questions you are looking for answers to. Focus on yourself, explore your intuitions, connect with your spirituality or simply let yourself be pervaded by discipline and self-control. If your goal is to detoxify your body, use it as an incentive to stay determined despite your hunger pangs.

If your fast allows you to drink only water, make sure you keep your body properly hydrated

Drink at least half a liter every two hours. Water fills the stomach, restores energy and dilutes digestive acids, which give rise to the feeling of hunger. While drinking is important, try not to exceed the recommended doses so as not to risk getting sick.

Some religious practices, such as the Islamic fasting rite, prohibit drinking anything from sunrise until sunset. In this scenario, it is essential to hydrate the body abundantly before and after fasting.

Keep yourself busy

Inactivity and boredom can make you want to eat, so try to distract yourself by doing something exciting that isn't physically strenuous. Reading, writing, meditating, slowly practicing yoga, working on the computer, walking in nature, watching television, or driving short distances are all great ways to keep yourself busy while fasting. Avoid activities that require a lot of energy, such as lifting weights, going to the gym or running long distances. As we have seen in previous chapters, exercising at an intense level forces you to burn a lot of calories, making you too hungry.

Try not to think about food. It is best to stay away from the kitchen, supermarket or food images and scents.

Be persistent

If you feel like giving up, remind yourself of your reasons for fasting. Show your discipline and tell yourself that hunger won't last forever. If you can stay determined, the ultimate reward will be far more satisfying than a little food.

Towards the end of your fast, you are likely to feel tired and exhausted. At that moment you will have to appeal to all your tenacity. Take a nap if you can, or let yourself be distracted by pictures or videos. An engaging action movie or video game can be of great help in this situation.

Break your fast at the scheduled time
Start eating slowly, being very careful not to overdo the quantities. Cut servings in half. In fact, it's extremely important not to eat as much as you normally would because the digestive system has been paused and still can't handle a massive amount of food. Avoid meat, fish or cheese, it is much better to break the fast by eating some fruit, vegetables or soup. It is also important to drink water and fruit juices.

Remember not to eat and not to drink too much or too fast. Start with an apple and a glass of water, then wait about ten minutes. At this point, you can eat a small portion of the soup and drink a glass of orange juice.

Break the fast over a period of about 30-60 minutes. Eating a lot right away could cause severe abdominal pain and dysentery, putting your health at serious risk. Do things gently and gradually.

Chapter 18

How to Fight the Urge to Eat

One of the most common difficulties women have when fasting is fighting the urge to eat. Oftentimes, this feeling is not associated with hunger itself but it has more to do with the habit of eating. In fact, most women are used to eating at least three meals a day and cutting back on this habit is not something easy to do.

While most books on intermittent fasting would tell you to just be strong and keep going, we know how difficult it can be not to break your fast when you are halfway through.

We want to do things differently and provide you with practical tips you can implement from the very beginning to fight the urge to eat.

Sometimes it can be helpful to learn how to control hunger. Being hungry all the time is frustrating and makes it difficult to maintain your ideal weight or stick to a diet plan. Many times it is not a question of real hunger or a physical need, but rather a manifestation of boredom. However, if your stomach is rumbling and you feel really hungry, there are a few things you can do to quickly reduce this feeling.

Do an inner analysis of your urge to eat
Whenever you feel hungry or have a desire to eat, pause for a few minutes and do a quick introspection. This way you can understand what is the best thing to do to deal with this feeling.
Many times you may feel hungry when in reality you are not really hungry. You may be bored, thirsty, agitated, stressed out, or just craving some tasty snack. Since there are a number of reasons that could lead you to eat that are not strictly related to a physical

need, it may be helpful to do this simple self-analysis first.

Take a few minutes to think about these questions and give yourself an honest answer.

Is your stomach "rumbling"? Do you have the impression that it is empty? When did you have your last meal or snack? Do you feel stressed, anxious or agitated? Are you bored? Ask yourself these questions to understand if you really need to eat.

If yours is a real physical need for food, you may consider interrupting the fast to eat a simple snack or wait until it's time for the next meal. You can also do some little tricks to quench your hunger for a while.

If yours isn't true hunger, find some other activity to distract yourself until the craving for food subsides.

Drink water or tea

Many times you may feel hungry and want to nibble or eat something, but in reality you are just thirsty. Symptoms of hunger and thirst are similar, so they can be easily confused.

Water can help fill your stomach and keep you from experiencing hunger pangs. In fact, when the stomach contains water, it sends a satiety signal to the brain.

If your stomach "complains", drink two full glasses or consider always carrying a bottle of water with you and drinking throughout the day, sipping from time to time. This way, among other things, you avoid getting dehydrated.

Hot or lukewarm water makes you feel even more full than water at room temperature. The taste and the warmth can convey the same feeling of "satisfaction" as a meal. Hot coffee or tea are also good options. However, if you have to pay attention to avoid calories because you are fasting, choose sugar-free drinks.

Brush your teeth

It's a really quick way to curb hunger in just a few seconds. You will have a lot less desire to have a snack if your teeth are clean.

The toothpaste leaves an intense flavor in the mouth, which immediately takes away the desire to eat. Also, many foods no longer taste the same way right after brushing your teeth.

Always carry a travel toothbrush if you get hungry during a long day away from home.

Find a particularly exciting activity to do

If you think you are hungry but don't experience typical hunger symptoms, then your craving may be triggered by other factors.

It is very common to want to eat out of boredom. In this case, immediately take your mind off the food by doing some other activity, so as to distract your mind for a while and overcome the desire to eat.

Go for a brisk walk, talk to a friend, read a good book, do some housework, or surf the internet. One study found that when you play tetris you feel less craving for food, so it might be a good time to indulge in some gaming.

Grab a bubble gum or eat a candy

Some studies have found that these "tricks" help reduce the feeling of hunger immediately.

This technique is believed to be so effective because the sensation of chewing or sucking on a tasty product sends the signal to the brain that the body is satisfied.

Choose sugar-free gums and candies, as they have to have zero calories to avoid breaking the fast. These products typically contain no calories and are great for stopping hunger pangs when dieting.

Do not skip breakfast

While there are several ways to get hunger under control quickly, a good breakfast can help reduce the feeling of hunger throughout the day.

If you skip breakfast, you will likely feel a lot more hungry for the next few hours. In addition to this, a study has shown that not having this first meal leads to eating more calories in the rest of the day. If you never eat breakfast, your body tends to increase the insulin response, promoting weight gain.

Research has found that eating a breakfast high in fat, protein and carbohydrates reduces hunger throughout the day.

When you are following an intermittent fasting protocol, we suggest having a healthy breakfast and fast for the rest of your day, not the other way around.

Here are some suggestions for a breakfast that can help you in this regard.

- Scrambled eggs with low-fat cheese and wholemeal toast;
- wholemeal flour waffles with peanut butter and fruit;
- oatmeal with dried and fresh fruit.

Eat adequate amounts of proteins

As we have seen in previous chapters, these substances perform several important tasks in the body, but at the same time help you feel full longer than other nutrients. Consuming protein also helps reduce cravings for sweet or high-fat foods.

Choose lean sources of protein (especially if you're particularly focused on weight loss) for each meal or snack. This way, you take them in adequate quantities for your needs, but you also feel satisfied and full throughout the day.

Among the various foods that provide lean protein you can consider: fish, poultry, lean beef, pork, eggs, low-fat dairy, legumes and tofu.

Make sure you eat protein foods within 30 minutes of exercising. Protein helps muscles absorb energy and develop. When following an intermittent fasting protocol, we advise you to exercise an hour after breaking your fast. In this way you have the time to eat something before your training session.

Choose foods that are rich in fiber

Several studies have found that people feel more satisfied and fuller by following a high-fiber diet than one that is deficient of this element.

There are several mechanisms that help induce the feeling of satiety with fibers. One of these is due to the fact that food that is rich in it has to be chewed a lot and takes longer to digest, thus increasing the sense of satiety. In addition, the fibers are voluminous, improving the feeling of fullness.

Vegetables, fruits, and whole grains are all high-fiber foods that typically leave you with a longer lasting sense of satisfaction than other foods.

Salads and vegetable soups are particularly valuable in this regard, as they are high in fiber and low in calories.

Another good thing about fiber is that it helps regulate blood sugar levels, keeping hunger pangs in check.

Satisfy your food cravings in a healthy way

There are probably many occasions when you are not really hungry, but want to have a snack or treat. A few concessions from time to time is fine, especially if you choose to satisfy this "craving" in a healthy way.

However, do not make it a habit to break your fast when you are not supposed to. Remember, creating a healthy intermittent fasting protocol means having the discipline to follow your plan.

There are several healthy alternatives to candy and salty, crunchy foods to calm the craving for food. Choose your snack wisely.

If you are craving for dessert, eat some fruit. An apple or orange provides fiber and vitamins, as well as some sugar to satisfy the need for sweetness.

If you feel craving for something more salty and crunchy, grab a small serving of salted nuts. Eat raw vegetables with hummus to satisfy the need for salty and crunchy.

However, once again we recommend you break the fast only if the urge to eat is too hard to fight. We encourage you to push yourself a bit as intermittent fasting can be a great mind exercise as well.

Chapter 19

How to Understand If You Are Truly Hungry or Not

During previous chapters we have mentioned different times how important it is to understand when you are too hungry to continue the fast and when you are just bored and have food cravings.

However, most women are so out of touch with their bodies that cannot properly distinguish these two very different situations. They have been conditioned over the years that each time their belly says something, it is important to answer by eating something. The following pages will give you a better understanding of the processes that you can put in place to understand if you are truly hungry or if you are just not accustomed to the feeling of intermittent fasting. Having a good grasp of this difference allows you to make better decisions and helps you stick to the protocol.

By practicing these tricks on a regular basis, you will develop your instinct and know when it is time to push it through and when it is better to have a snack.

It can be quite difficult to distinguish physical from emotional hunger. This is especially true if you are not very familiar with recognizing the signals your body is sending you. Physical hunger typically comes on gradually and subsides after eating a meal. However, some women often tend to eat even when they don't really need to eat. In this case, it is emotional hunger that leads to eating when you are in certain psychological states: stress, boredom, anxiety, happiness or even depression. Therefore, understanding hunger and knowing how it affects the body can help distinguish between a symptom of a physiological need and an emotional problem. This chapter is intended to give you some tips to learn about your body, hunger levels, and how to avoid the temptation to eat when in reality it is not yet time to feed.

Rank your hunger level on a scale of 1 to 10

This method can help you figure out what to do. It should give you an idea on whether to eat a snack and break the fast or wait until the next scheduled meal. Try to establish hunger from level 1 (almost faint from hunger) to level 10 (completely full, almost nauseous). If your hunger level is around 3 or 4, it may be time to eat even if your intermittent fasting protocol says not to do it. If your next meal isn't scheduled within a couple of hours, have a snack. If, on the other hand, you are expected to eat within an hour or so, try to hold on until you sit down at the table.

In theory, you shouldn't go to extremes: neither go hungry at level 1, nor overdo it and eat until level 10. Try to stick to the 4-7 values.

It is normal and predictable to feel hungry before a meal and even just before going to sleep in the evening.

Take the apple test

This is a simple test that can help you figure out if you are having a physical or emotional hunger attack. Typically, psychological hunger is the need and desire to eat something from a particular food group (such as carbohydrates) or a specific food (such as chocolate cake). Physical hunger, on the other hand, is satisfied with a wide variety of foods.

Ask yourself if you want to eat a snack even if it was an apple, a raw carrot or a salad.

If so, eat an apple (another fruit or vegetable) or another healthy, planned snack that really satisfies your physical hunger.

If not, you probably need to satisfy an emotional hunger and not a physical hunger.

If you have determined that it is psychological hunger, this is the right time to go for a walk or take a 10-minute break and reflect on the reason for your upset.

Observe yourself

Before eating any meal or snack, take a minute or two to analyze yourself internally. By doing this, you can understand your true level of hunger and desire to eat.

Evaluate various aspects such as the level of hunger. Do you feel undernourished? Are you full instead? Do you feel satisfied?

Take note of the physical signs of hunger. Your stomach may "grumble", you may feel empty or feel hunger cramps, if it is a real need to eat.

If you feel the desire to eat something without a real physical need, analyze your emotional state. Are you bored? Have you had a stressful day at work? Do you feel tired or exhausted? Many times these moods induce a feeling of "hunger" when in reality it is not a real physical need to eat food.

Drink enough water

Aim to drink adequate amounts of fluids each day. Usually, it is recommended to drink about 8 glasses or almost 2 liters of water. This is just a general recommendation. In fact, you could drink a little more or a little less. Proper hydration helps you lose weight, but it's also important for managing hunger levels throughout the day.

If you are thirsty or a little dehydrated, you may experience a feeling of hunger. If you don't drink properly every day, dehydration can trigger hunger, which can cause you to eat more food or more often than you need to.

Keep a bottle of water on hand at all times and pay attention to how much you drink each day. Also, try to drink just before a meal to calm hunger and reduce food intake.

Wait 10 to 15 minutes and see what happens

Emotional hunger can come on suddenly, but it can disappear just as quickly, unlike the physical need to eat. If you take 10-15 minutes of distraction from the situation you are experiencing, you may find that your food cravings and emotional urge to eat are reduced and you are able to control them much more easily.

By waiting a few minutes, the craving for food does not completely disappear, but it subsides enough to be able to overcome it with willpower.

Try telling yourself that during this time you can re-evaluate your ideas about eating some specific food or snack. Engage in another activity, but go back to considering breaking the fast if the need is still there.

Empty the kitchen

If you have a fridge or pantry full of unhealthy foods that tempt you, it can be easier to give in to emotional hunger. If you know that you can easily have a packet of crackers or a bag of chips when you are bored or stressed, do not keep these foods at home, so as not to be tempted when you are overwhelmed by these feelings; by doing so, you can eat less if you are not really hungry.

Take an hour or two to scan the kitchen. Check the pantry, fridge, freezer, and cupboards at home where you keep food. Put all the foods and snacks that make you want to eat on the table and examine them to decide which ones to keep and which ones to discard.

Donate any still packaged items to the food counter or church if you don't want to throw them in the trash.

Make a promise to yourself not to buy tempting but unhealthy snacks anymore, so that your kitchen and home are healthy environments.

Get away from food

Sometimes, the very fact of being in the same room as your favorite foods or some food you crave to eat makes it harder to ignore the urge to fill your belly. If you are in a place in your home or office that increases your desire to eat, get away. Take the time and space to clear your mind of the need for some "rewarding treats".

Take a walk for 15 minutes if you can. Distract your mind and bring attention to other thoughts that are not related to nutrition.

Sometimes, some people feel the urge to have some nighttime snacks. Instead of staying awake, go to bed. In this way, you stay away from the kitchen and aren't tempted to unwittingly eat in front of the TV. If you are not tired, read a good book or magazine until you are sleepy enough to fall asleep.

Make a list of the things you can do instead of eating

This "trick" can distract your mind from food cravings and help you manage emotional hunger. Make a quick list of activities that you enjoy or that distract you enough to take your thoughts away from food. Here are some ideas-

- Clean the cupboards or rearrange the junk drawer;
- Take a walk;

- Engage in your favorite hobby;
- Read a book or magazine;
- Play a game.

Eat a small portion of the food you just can't resist

Sometimes, the need or desire to eat can overwhelm you uncontrollably. Even if you get distracted and try to reduce the craving for food, it can be very intense. If that is the case, some experts recommend consuming a small, controlled portion of that food you crave to eat.

By limiting yourself to a small portion, you can reduce your food cravings, but at the same time allow yourself the pleasure of eating something tasty.

Make sure it's a very small portion. Read the nutrition label and measure the appropriate amount, put the rest away and slowly enjoy your dose so you can enjoy all the flavor.

Please, note that this practice still counts as breaking the fast. So do not use it unless the craving is unbearable.

Keep a diary

It is a great tool for raising awareness and managing emotional hunger. You can use it to understand where and when you eat, which types of foods give you the most comfort, and which ones you want to eat most often.

Purchase a food diary or download a smartphone app. Monitor as many days as possible - both during the week and on the weekend. Many people eat differently on weekends, so it's important to take note of both situations.

Also take into account any feelings or moods you experience when you eat. This can help you learn more about the emotions that cause you to eat certain foods.

Talk to a qualified dietician or behavioral therapist

These health professionals can help you manage emotional hunger. If you are having trouble keeping your appetite in check or you see that it is putting your health at risk, it is a wise idea to keep in touch with a doctor.

The dietician is an experienced nutritionist who can help you understand emotional hunger, explain true physical hunger to you, and can point you to alternative food options.

The behavioral therapist will help you understand why you are feeling emotional hunger and can give you some tips to change your reactions and behavior in the face of certain triggers.

Find a support group

Regardless of your health goal, a support group plays an important role in achieving long-term positive results. This is even more true when hunger is emotional. Having this kind of support when you're feeling sad or stressed can help you lift your mood without the need for food.

Whether it's your spouse, family, friends, or coworkers, a support group can motivate and encourage you as you progress.

Also look for an online support group or people who gather for this purpose in your city. Email new friends who share your long-term goals and tell them about your intermittent fasting protocol.

Having someone by your side will make all the difference in the world.

Chapter 20

Intermittent Fasting and Juicing

Some women might find juicing an interesting way to take intermittent fasting to the next level. While in the long run we feel it is too stressful for the body and the mind, if done for a couple of days every month it can truly help you lose weight and purify your body.

In this chapter we dive a bit deeper into this topic and try to understand how to go about juicing. As you will soon discover, juicing while on an intermittent fasting protocol has some interesting and particular details that should be known before beginning this practice.

A juice-only fast is ideal for ridding the body of toxins and promoting weight loss. Plus, it's a healthier type of detox than simple water-based fasting, especially for those who aren't used to it. In fact, the body still receives large amounts of vitamins and nutrients. This chapter will teach you to follow fasting safely and effectively, but you should definitely talk to your doctor about fasting before embarking on it.

Set a goal

Those women who are already experienced with fasting can choose a juice-based diet that lasts approximately 3 weeks. However, if this is your first time, it is recommended to start with a smaller, more manageable goal, such as three days. Fasting can be difficult, both physically and mentally, so it may be easier to start with a reachable goal. It is better to successfully complete a short fast than to falter in the middle of a long one.

A 3-day fast is actually an integral part of a program that lasts 5 days. In fact, you have to calculate 24 hours to get the body accustomed to fasting and another 24 to return to your usual eating habits.

If this is your first fast, it may be helpful to convince a friend to go through the process together. You can motivate each other, and a bit of competitiveness will keep you from giving in to temptation.

Go shopping at the supermarket

For a juice fast, you need large amounts of fresh fruits and vegetables, probably more than you think. It is very important to buy organic agricultural products, not treated with pesticides. The idea of doing such a diet is to get rid of the toxins you have in your body, not introduce any more.

Fill up on oranges, lemons, limes, tomatoes, spinach, kale, celery, carrots, cucumbers, apples, grapes, blueberries, beets, garlic and ginger root.

If possible, you should also get good quality spring water, bottled by a company that uses food-grade plastic or glass containers. Drinking lots of water is an integral part of the diet.

Invest in a good juicer

Having a quality juicer is essential to performing this fast, since it maximizes the amount of juice you get from fruits and vegetables, and saves you time and effort in preparation and cleaning. Make sure the juicer has a power of at least 700 watts, so that it can effectively squeeze any type of fresh fruit you introduce. You should also look for a juicer that has as few parts as possible to assemble and disassemble, as this will speed up the process.

Buying a new juicer can be a considerable expense, but the investment is worth it, especially if you plan to do this fast regularly, integrating it into your lifestyle. Generally, you have to spend around 200 dollars to buy a good juicer, but it could last you 15-20 years.

It is not possible to replace the juicer with the blender to accomplish this fast. If you use the blender, you will end up with a smoothie, not a juice. A smoothie retains the fiber of fruit and vegetables. While this is usually good, you don't need fiber while doing a juice fast. This is because the body uses too much energy when digesting them, the energy it needs to get rid of toxins.

Decide when to do the juice fast

Timing is an important aspect of every fast. You need to make sure you have enough time in the morning to make juices and don't plan on activities that require a lot of energy while fasting, especially if it's your first time. Remember it lasts 3-5 days. Many people who decide to try this method without ever having done it before plan it over the weekend, from Friday to Sunday, when they can stay at home for long periods of time.

Some suffer from headaches and low vitality when following this path (while others report having higher energy levels than usual). Additionally, you may feel the need to take a mid-afternoon nap to conserve energy.

You should also remember that juice fasting stimulates the elimination of toxins from the body, so the body will need to get rid of waste frequently. For this reason, it is best to stay close to a bathroom while fasting.

Prepare your body for juice fasting

Before the actual fast begins, which will last for 3 days, you need to remember that you need 24 hours to prepare your body for the experience. You can do this by eating only raw fruits and vegetables in the 24 hours before fasting. If you like, you can get your body used to it by drinking only juices for breakfast and lunch, and then prepare a solid dinner of salad or other raw fruit and vegetables.

Some people also recommend clearing the body with a purgative (a natural laxative) or enema before the fast begins, but this is optional and we do not recommend it for beginners.

Make enough fresh juice every morning

If you have enough time when you wake up, you can save yourself a good deal of effort throughout the day by preparing all the juices you will drink during the day. Then, keep them in the refrigerator until you are ready to consume them. Alternatively, you can simply prepare the fruit and vegetables you intend to use for each juice, and place them in airtight bags in the refrigerator until you can make the juice.

Experiment with different combinations of fruits and vegetables to get tasty and unusual results. Try to think carefully about the flavors that would work well when mixed; in this way, drinking juices will be a pleasure rather than an obligation.

When doing a juice fast, you should try to keep a ratio of 20:80 between fruit-based and vegetable-based juices. Fruit juices actually contain a lot of sugars, which are more difficult for the body to assimilate, so maybe limit their consumption in the morning. For lunch and dinner, on the other hand, prefer vegetable-based juices.

Drink as many juices as you want throughout the day

This juice detox shouldn't make you starve. The body needs the vitamins and nutrients in the juice to keep you active and perform that important task of eliminating toxins. For this reason, there is no limit to the amount of juice you should drink over the course of a day. Whenever you feel hungry or thirsty, drink a smoothie. You should consume at least 4 servings a day.

If you have read the previous chapters, you know that this is a big difference if compared to the standard intermittent fasting protocol.

If you want to do your juice-based detox for weight loss, you should still avoid limiting your juice intake. With this fast, the body is already deprived of enough calories; reducing the juice intake will therefore send it into survival mode, and this will lead him to retain more weight. So, stick to a minimum of 4 drinks per day.

Drink lots of water

Keeping yourself hydrated is extremely important during a juice-based fast. In fact, water helps you eliminate toxins from the body, and allows you to regain hydration after the purifying action. Plus, it allows you to keep hunger pangs in check. You should aim to consume at least 500ml of water with each juice; you can either dilute the juice 50% with water or ingest the 2 drinks separately, one after the other. You should also drink additional water in between juices. Drinking herbal tea is another great way to get more water, as long as you prefer the healthy, theine-free versions.

Do not train too hard

While fasting, a little bit of physical activity allows you to distract your mind from hunger pangs, and will help boost your metabolism. A short walk outdoors or some simple yoga poses are all it takes to stay healthy, but avoid exercises that are more vigorous than these, as they may make you feel weak.

Follow the juicing schedule for the next 48 hours, drinking as much juice and water as you like. If you run out of fresh fruits and vegetables, you need to go back to the supermarket. You should also keep experimenting with different recipes to make the juices varied and interesting.

Don't lose your focus

As enthusiastic as you feel at the start of the purification, you will surely find yourself facing temptations and testing your willpower over the course of these 3 days. You will become more sensitive to smells and solid foods will seem inviting like never before. Stay strong and remember why you decided to start a juice fast in the first place. You are getting rid of harmful substances that have accumulated in the body for so many years and are losing weight at the same time. You will feel much better in the end, both physically and mentally, and appreciate the satisfaction of successfully completing your first juice detox.

Some women like the fasting process and claim to experience a net increase in energy instead of a drain. Maybe, you will be one of these lucky women.

Try not to think about fasting by engaging in relaxing and rejuvenating activities, such as meditation, reading, stretching and manual projects. By not having to plan your day between meals, you will have much more free time at your disposal.

Take a day to get your body used to the end of the fast. This day will be similar to the day before the detox: you will only eat salads and fruit. Consume small portions so you don't overload your stomach and digestive system.

Gradually return to normal food consumption
After letting your body get used to it, you can progressively return to your usual diet by introducing foods such as eggs, dairy products, rice and whole grains, lean meats. However, you should try to refrain

from consuming processed foods to avoid undermining the good work done during detox.

Eating pizza or other processed foods right after you finish your juice fast is not a good idea, and this could also make you feel sick.

Think about introducing a 24-hour weekly juice fast into your intermittent fasting routine. Detoxifying your body with juices once a week will help you maintain the purifying level you have reached with this experience. In fact, it's pretty simple to implement, because you can divide these 24 hours over 2 days. The night before, start with an early dinner, then eat nothing else for the rest of the evening. Sleep for 8 hours, then drink juice for breakfast and lunch the next day. Finally, you can have a solid meal at dinner time, when the purification is complete-

Next time, try fasting longer
Once you have successfully completed a 3-day juice fast, you can take it one step further to make regular detoxes last longer. If you want, commit to completing a 7 or even 14 day juice fast. As daunting as it may

seem, many women who have some experience with intermittent fasting argue that juice fasting actually gets easier when periods without solid food get longer. The body gets used to not feeling hungry on its own, because it recognizes that it is getting all the nutrients it needs from the juices.

Either way, be careful. With longer fasts, the body begins to eliminate toxins through the skin and lungs, and you may find that you have a strange or unpleasant smell.

If you are juice fasting longer, you should include protein and iron supplements in your juices to get more energy and avoid becoming anemic. These supplements are available in drug stores and health food stores.

We highly recommend introducing juice fasting into your regular intermittent fasting protocol. However, if you are just starting out, our advice is not to overdo. If you find yourself struggling to keep a healthy intermittent fasting regimen, stick to that before introducing this variation.

Chapter 21

Practical Tips to Complete a Fast

In this chapter we are going to discuss some practical tips that will help you complete your fast without feeling overwhelmed by the different feelings and emotions you might experience.

There are many reasons why people choose to fast. Your fast may be designed to make you lose weight or detoxify you, or be part of a spiritual practice. Whatever your reasons, facing and overcoming a fast may not be easy. Don't worry though, with the right preparation, determination and self-care you will be able to reach your goal.

As we have mentioned time and time again, before embarking on a fast, it is always good to consult a doctor. Changing your diet drastically will have a noticeable effect on your body, especially if you have some underlying disease that could get worse with fasting (for example, diabetes). Whatever your health situation is, it is always advisable to consult your doctor before starting a fast.

Many people decide to fast for religious reasons rather than in an attempt to lose weight, detox or regain their physical shape. However, it should be noted that all religions, including Islam, Catholicism and Judaism, allow an exception to be made for all those whose health does not allow fasting in safe conditions. Nonetheless, we think that if you are reading this it is because you are interested in losing weight, not in following some spiritual or religious practices.

Before starting to fast, hydrate your body properly

Without ingesting food, the human body appears to be able to survive for weeks, or in one documented case even for months, but without water it will quickly collapse. Being made up of about 60% water, in order to function, our organism and each of its cells have a considerable need. Without water, most people would die within three days. As you have learned so far, there are different forms of fasting, but in any case, water should never be completely denied. During the month of Islamic Ramadan, believers are forbidden to drink water for long periods of time, but whatever your form of fasting it is important to prepare your body for a nutritional deficiency by "super-hydrating" it in advance.

During the days leading up to the fast, drink plenty of water on a regular basis. Also, before the last meal before fasting begins, take at least 2 liters of moisturizing fluids.

To avoid the risk of dehydrating the body, also avoid foods that are very salty or high in sugar, such as sweet and savory snacks and fast food.

Limit your caffeine intake

Many of the drinks we consume every day, such as coffee, tea and energy or carbonated drinks, contain large doses of caffeine, a substance capable of changing our mood and causing a real addiction. If you are used to taking caffeine and suddenly cutting it out of your diet, you will most likely experience withdrawal symptoms. When you eat normally, these symptoms can go almost unnoticed, but during a fast, even a short one (even for a single day), the signs of crisis can be strongly felt.

Common symptoms of caffeine withdrawal include headache, fatigue, anxiety, irritability, sadness, and difficulty concentrating.

To avoid these unwanted side effects, work to break the habit early by gradually reducing your caffeine intake in the weeks leading up to the start of the intermittent fasting cycle.

Cut down on smoking

If you are addicted to tobacco, you may have more difficulty than having to do without caffeine. Nonetheless, being able to quit smoking is even more important than giving up caffeine. By smoking on an empty stomach, your body and health will be hit hard and you may feel nauseous and dizzy. Tobacco consumption during an intermittent fasting protocol increases blood pressure, heart rate and lowers the skin temperature of the fingers and toes.

If you are having a hard time quitting smoking, even temporarily, see your doctor for a more effective strategy or read books about it. There are some pretty useful guides out there.

Choose foods that are high in carbohydrates
The term "carbohydrate" itself means "carbon rich in water". Unlike proteins and fats, carbohydrates bind to water and allow the body to stay hydrated for longer periods of time. This quality of carbohydrates is very important when preparing for a fast. During the weeks leading up to it, consume large amounts of carbohydrate-rich foods so your body can keep its water reserves tight. We advise you try some of the following foods before and during your intermittent fasting protocol.

- Bread and pasta prepared with multigrain, wholemeal flours and different types of cereals;
- Starchy vegetables (potatoes);
- Vegetables (lettuce, broccoli, asparagus, carrots);
- Fruits (tomatoes, strawberries, apples, berries, oranges, grapes and bananas).

Keep the mealsize under control

In the days leading up to your fast, you may be tempted to overeat to fill up on vitamins, nutrients, and calories. The basic idea will be to fill up in advance to be able to last as long as possible without eating. In fact, however, ingesting large quantities of food will only accustom your body to large meals and, once you stop eating, you will actually feel even more hungry. It is also advisable to vary the meal times every day so that the body does not get used to receiving food at specific times.

Before starting the fast, have a large meal, but don't binge. After eating high-carb foods for days, many women choose to have a "last" protein-rich meal to feel satisfied for a longer period of time and to enter the fast more easily.

Before your final meal, don't forget to take a substantial amount of moisturizing fluids to facilitate a smooth transition to fasting.

Keep busy

Hunger is a primary feeling related to the whole body and, if left free to do, can take control of the mind.

Being obsessed with it is the quickest way to failing to overcome fasting. Distract yourself as much as possible by constantly keeping yourself busy.

Engage in light, enjoyable activities, such as chatting with friends or reading a good book.

Taking care of those chores and tasks that you usually put off is another way to effectively keep yourself busy. When the aim is to be able to distract you from hunger, even the hypothesis of cleaning the whole house may not seem so bad!

When you are following an intermittent fasting protocol, reduce the amount of exercise you do

In some cases, based on the reasons and nature of the fast, more vigorous activities may not be recommended or permitted. If you are doing "intermittent fasting," where you fast regularly for a short period of time every given number of days, you are more likely to lose weight. Training a carbohydrate-deficient body means forcing it to burn fat to sustain itself; for many this could be a primary goal. However, note that, at the same time, your body will also begin to burn proteins and muscle mass. The best thing you can do is exercise at a slow pace and avoid exhaustion with a cardio workout.

If you intend to fast for a long time, avoid very tiring activities. Those who follow intermittent fasting simply abstain from food for short periods of time. Even if you have to avoid cardio training, it is good for them to exercise because they will soon give their bodies new fuel. If you intend to fast for several days, however, it is best to avoid any energy-intensive activities. Otherwise you would otherwise feel much more tired than when you do them by feeding normally. Fasting for an extended period, rather than intermittently, means not providing your body with any fuel for a long time. This is why we always recommend women over 50 years of age to follow an intermittent fasting routine, rather than doing prolonged fasting.

Get enough rest
When you sleep, you think you are calm and relaxed, but in reality your body is working to take care of itself. The night's rest gives it the opportunity to repair muscles, form memories, regulate its growth and

appetite through hormones. When you fast, lack of food can cause problems with concentration. Regular naps throughout the day have been shown to improve alertness, mood, and mental sharpness.

Get your body at least 8 hours of sleep each night and take regular naps throughout the day while on an intermittent fasting protocol.

Hang out with other women who are fasting like you

Those who are fasting for spiritual reasons will be facilitated because many of their friends and acquaintances belonging to the same place of worship will be doing the same. Even if you are fasting for health reasons or to purify yourself, it is still advisable to seek the company of a friend who does the same. Being surrounded by people who are on the same path as you will allow you not to feel alone in this experience. Whatever your goals, commit to motivating and empowering each other to achieve them.

Don't talk about food while on an intermittent fasting protocol

Don't put yourself in uncomfortable situations where you might feel sorry for yourself. Even in the presence of other people like you who are facing a fast, do not allow the conversation to turn on the lack and desire for food. By obsessing over the thought of food you will end up not being able to stop thinking about it and you will risk taking a false step as soon as you find yourself alone. Instead of describing what you are missing, develop your conversations in positive terms, for example by analyzing the many benefits you will derive from this experience. Alternatively, you can talk about something completely different, such as the movie you have just seen or a current situation you are dealing with.

As long as the fast is in progress, avoid accepting any invitation involving a meal, even from friends. Even if they didn't tempt you to break your fast by eating in front of your eyes, they would force you to have a difficult and painful experience.

Describe your intermittent fasting protocol in a journal

Even when you can count on the support of a friend to help you stay responsible, sharing some frustrating moments and feelings may not be easy. A diary will then allow you to keep your thoughts private and give a free space to your emotions. If you want, in the future, you can re-read your words to perform a thorough analysis. You can write in your diary as you normally would, recounting simple daily events, or choose to focus exclusively on fasting-related issues. Either way, many of your intimate thoughts are likely to be related to your intermittent fasting protocol in some way.

Don't censor yourself! Even if you are following an intermittent fasting protocol for religious reasons, do not hold back from expressing your possible desire to end the fast. With the simple act of writing down your thoughts, you will be able to cope with them better and let them escape from your mind, and stop feeling obsessed with them.

Plan to break your fast

However hungry you may be at the end of your fast, it will be important to resist the temptation to binge at the earliest opportunity. During an intermittent fasting protocol, the body implements mechanisms that allow it to adapt to the lack of food by slowing the production of those enzymes that facilitate digestion. By binging immediately after stopping it, you will force your body to handle a quantity of food that it is currently unable to process, putting you at risk of stomach cramps, nausea and vomiting. During the last few days of your intermittent fasting protocol, you will need to develop a plan that will allow you to easily resume a regular diet.

To start reintroducing fluids, start drinking fruit juices and eating fresh fruit

Of course, in case you have continued to drink only juices, drinking more of them will not exactly "break" your fast. For those who have only been drinking water though, drinking and eating high water content juices and fruits is the best way to allow the body to return to normal. As we fast, our stomach tends to shrink in size, therefore, by drinking juices and eating fruit initially, we may be able to feel satisfied quickly.

You can follow the tips discussed in the chapter dedicated to juice fasting to see how to properly reintroduce fluids after a long intermittent fasting protocol.

Facilitates the transition to small solid meals
Instead of preparing a single large meal with which to end your fast, have snacks or small meals spread throughout the day. To avoid prematurely overloading your sleeping digestive system, stop eating at the first signs of satiety. Initially it is good to focus only on foods with a high water content such as the following.
- Soups and broths
- Vegetables
- Raw fruit
- Yogurt

Chew your food carefully
When breaking a fast, chewing has two main tasks. First, it prevents you from eating the meal too fast,

and in this regard it is good to note that the brain takes about 20 minutes to process the information it receives from the stomach and realize that this organ is full. Eating too quickly leads to binge eating, which is dangerous when coming out of an intermittent fasting protocol. The second benefit of proper chewing is the breaking down of food into smaller, more easily digestible pieces.

Make an effort to chew each bite about 15 times.

Drink a glass of water before your meal and sip another while you eat to slow down the rate of ingestion. Take a quick sip between bites.

Take probiotics

Probiotics are "good bacteria" that spread naturally in the mouth, intestines and vagina. They promote efficient digestion and are therefore valid allies when we break an intermittent fasting protocol. Choose those foods that contain active lactobacillus cultures, including yogurt, sauerkraut, and miso. Alternatively, you can help your digestion by taking a probiotic supplement in capsule, tablet or powder form.

Listen to your body

Whatever information you read in this book about the best way to break an intermittent fasting protocol, your own body will let you know what it feels ready for. If after reintroducing fruit and vegetables you feel stomach cramps or feel the need to vomit, don't force yourself any further! Go back to eating only fruit and drinking only juice for another meal, or for a whole day. Allow your body to progress at its own pace. Soon you will be able to digest even a heavier meal or heavier foods again without suffering from any side effects.

Chapter 22

Intermittent Fasting and Sleep

When starting an intermittent fasting protocol, some women might see a negative reaction in their sleep pattern. It is absolutely normal, but we understand how it can affect your mood and overall ability to keep on going with your fasting when things get difficult.

There are a couple of tips and tricks that you can implement that can assure you are well rested even during an intense intermittent fasting protocol. This chapter is going to dive deeper into this topic and tell you everything you need to know to make the most out of your sleep.

When your sleep is constantly interrupted or you just can't fall asleep easily, it can happen that you are severely tempted to resort to sleeping pills. Still, sleeping pills don't prepare you to sleep properly without them, and they tend to leave many women over 50 tired in the morning, as well as addicted to heavy and prolonged intake of these pills. They are more like a shortcut unable to produce any change, especially in the way we eat.

So, can you sleep without sleeping pills? There are many solutions involving food (and drinks) that can be used to sleep better. Here's how to be generous with your belly so it leaves you alone when you want to sleep.

Find out about the foods and drinks that may make it worse for you to fall asleep
Before choosing foods and drinks that can help you sleep better, it is vital to remove food sources that may be preventing you from falling asleep or sleeping as you would like. The worst are caffeine, alcohol and sugar. The following foods need to be slathered into your diet so you don't deprive yourself of sleep.

- **Caffeine**. Caffeine is present in coffee, tea, chocolate, cola, certain energy drinks and derived foods and medicines. The amount of caffeine in each element varies based on the strength and type of food. In general, it is best to stop drinking or consuming caffeinated products at least five hours before bedtime. The older you are, the more sensitive you are to caffeine, which is able to remove sleepiness, make you stay awake longer than necessary, bring fatigue, heartburn, tremors, etc., and can end up depriving you of deep restorative sleep.

- **Alcohol**. Although alcohol can make you feel sleepy initially, it upsets your sleep while you sleep! Alcohol can reduce REM sleep and the duration of sleep, as well as lead you to sleep more superficially and wake up often during the night. And for beauty lovers, alcohol causes noticeable bags under the eyes!

- **Sugar**. Sugar is found in a broad spectrum of processed, natural and cooked foods. Any form of sugar can interrupt sleep if you take too much. The problem with sugar is the spike in blood sugar it creates, followed by its subsequent collapse; the frequency of this process reduces our energy levels and leaves us fatigued; our night cycles are also disturbed by the low energy level caused by an excessive amount of sugar.

Avoid hard-to-digest foods

What causes indigestion in one person may easily not produce the same effect in another. The point is to know the causes of indigestion and manage them. Some of the more common causes are the following.

- Any food you are intolerant to (those you are allergic to should not be consumed at all) - the most common intolerances are gluten, dairy, chocolate or sugar;
- Large meals before bed. When you don't give your body enough time to break down food and lie down immediately after eating, indigestion symptoms are likely to arise. Stop eating calorie dense foods at least five hours before going to bed. A light and healthy diet not only takes care of weight but also reduces the risk of sleep apnea.

- Onions, beans and peppers can cause indigestion in vulnerable people.

Choose foods that stabilize your energy when following an intermittent fasting protocol

These are foods that allow you to avoid extreme levels of blood suger, while still providing you with the energy you need during the day. Normal energy levels avoid irritability, fatigue, stress and exhaustion; they also improve mood and facilitate sleep making you feel more calm, rested and balanced. Foods that stabilize energy levels include the following.

- Foods rich in proteins: lean meats, cheeses, natural yogurt, eggs, fish, wholemeal bread, dried legumes, beans, lentils, nuts, seeds, etc. they are stable sources of protein that give you energy.
- Chromium-rich foods: Chromium will help your body overcome low sugar levels. It can be found in shellfish, cooked beans and cheese.
- Fresh fruit: it is better than snacks. By consuming it, you will have the benefit of fiber, nutrients and a slow energy release, so avoid replacing it with juices, nuts or desserts. Apples

and pears relax the digestive system the most, especially while following an intermittent fasting protocol.

Drink lots of water

Water gives life and is devoid of substances that waste energy. In addition, it provides an important aid to good digestion. Try to drink two liters of water (about eight glasses) a day.

Increase the intake of foods high in tryptophan

Tryptophan helps synthesize proteins, being an amino acid and an essential chemical element. It is found in meat, fish, vegetables and eggs, and its consumption in the hours preceding sleep will release melatonin and serotonin, which can promote sleep. It increases the feeling of sleepiness, lowers the level of spontaneous nocturnal awakenings and helps to increase the amount of restful sleep.

It is recommended to have a main meal about four hours before bed, making sure it has complex carbohydrates and foods rich in tryptophan. Of course, have a meal in the evening only if it is prescribed by your intermittent fasting protocol.

If you are hungry before going to sleep, choose a snack high in tryptophan, but make sure you spend at least an hour between meals and sleep, to allow for adequate digestion.

Some snacks to consider before bed are the following.
- Dried fruit and tofu;
- Cheese and crackers;
- Milk and cereals;
- Apple pie with ice cream;
- Biscuits with cereals and raisins;
- Banana and wholemeal bread toast;
- Bread and peanut butter;

Choose foods with a natural relaxing effect
Calcium and magnesium relax the mind, so foods rich in these elements will increase your chances of sleeping well. Additionally, there are some foods known for sedative properties like the following.
- Lettuce. It contains a substance linked to opium, as well as atropine, capable of preventing cramps. Lettuce can be drizzled with a pinch of lemon and drunk before bed - much better than sleeping pills!

- Complex carbohydrates. They contain serotonin, which promotes sleep; this category includes pasta, brown rice and oatmeal.
- Mandarin juice. It contains bromine, a relaxing substance.

Pay attention to the glycemic index of foods

As we have mentioned in previous chapters as well, the glycemic index plays an important role while following an intermittent fasting protocol. The GI is a food unit of measurement that refers to the processing speed of the food we ingest. Slower processed food keeps us full for longer and tends to be generally healthier, so it has a low GI. Low GI foods maintain better sugar levels, helping us feel better, more balanced and rested throughout the day. Before bed, a day of low GI foods leaves you naturally tired and ready to sleep. Low GI foods include the following ingredients.

- Wholemeal bread, pasta, rice, sweet potatoes, mixed green salad or lightly sautéed vegetables.
- Dried pulses, lentils, and beans are excellent low GI foods.

The more processed a food is, the higher its GI will be.

Try drinking herbal tea, which is guaranteed to promote sleep. There are many herbs that promote sleep. When transformed into herbal tea via infusion or decoction, they can induce drowsiness. We suggest you drink one of the following types of herbal tea.

- Chamomile: in sachets or home grown and dried. Adding honey or ginger can improve the flavor.
- Verbena: Also known as lemon grass, it helps you sleep.
- Lemon balm: "lemon" member of the mint family, which helps you sleep.
- Passiflora (passion flower): this herb is relaxing. It can be effective against insomnia and anxiety; follow the directions on the package. If you have an irritable stomach, try this tea three times a day.
- Lime: use dried flowers to make tea.

Increase the intake of vitamins and minerals to improve sleep

If you're not already following a healthy intermittent fasting protocol, your nutrient levels may be low. There are many vitamins and minerals important for a good night's sleep, including vitamin B, calcium, magnesium, vitamin C, and chromium.

Taking vitamins and minerals through a healthy diet is always preferable, but sometimes supplements are the only way to get the necessary dose of a specific nutrient; consult a doctor for more in-depth advice.

In some countries it is possible to take melatonin, a hormone considered by some to be a stimulant for sleep during the most intense intermittent fasting protocols. However, take into account the meager scientific evidence about the benefits of melatonin supplements for sleep, and you will inevitably reduce the amount of melatonin your body produces. It is probably best to leave these products to older women, whose melatonin production is physiologically declining.

We understand the importance of sleeping well, especially while on an intermittent fasting protocol. If you follow these tips we are sure you are going to feel much better before going to bed, which is something that will ensure you a good night of deep sleep.

Our advice is to stay away from sleeping pills as much as possible. A healthy intermittent fasting protocol incorporates all the strategic elements needed to sleep well.

Chapter 23

Intermittent Fasting and Supplements

Supplements play an important role when it comes to following an intermittent fasting protocol in the best possible way. In fact, many women think that it is sufficient to eat good foods when breaking the fast to stay healthy. Research shows that this could not be farther from the truth. In fact, studies have shown time and time again that women that follow an intermittent fasting protocol experience some nutritional deficits even if their diet is on point.

In this chapter, we are going to give you all the information you need to start supplementing your nutrition with healthy products that can help you lose weight, keep it off and be healthy at the same time.

Let's start by giving a clear and simple definition of what food supplements are. Food supplements are products that are used to supplement the normal diet.

Therefore, they are not medicines, although they too are subject to strict regulation by the current legislation.

The food supplements market is extremely broad, it includes products suitable for the most varied needs and containing ingredients of different types. In no case, however, these products can be considered as an alternative to healthy and balanced lifestyle habits and even less as a remedy to stem or repair the damage caused by the incorrect habits mentioned above.

Therefore, the correct approach for the right use of food supplements, involves first of all the knowledge of these products (what are they? What is their purpose?), and secondly the ability of the consumers to understand when they can freely take similar products. Another important thing is to understand when it is necessary to consult a doctor before taking supplements. Although they are not drugs, in fact, even food supplements can give rise to side effects and can have various contraindications. For this reason, in case of doubts and in the presence of pathologies, disorders or particular conditions (for example, menopause), the consultation of the doctor is essential.

Food supplements can be formulated in the form of tablets, effervescent tablets, capsules, gummy candies, powders (in containers with measuring cups, or in single-dose sachets) and solutions (generally, in single-dose vials).

These are free sale products, marketed both in pharmacies and parapharmacies (including online) and in herbalist's shops, supermarkets and other shops, both physical and online.

What are Food Supplements used for?

Food supplements are used to supplement the normal diet in cases where there is a deficit of nutrients, for reduced intake, or for increased needs.

Depending on the type, food supplements can also be used to support diets (for example, adjuvant supplements for low-calorie diets, supplements for vegetarians or vegans) or other treatments, as well as they can be used to support the body's functions in particularly intense or stressful periods (e.g. sports supplements, memory supplements, etc.). In this regard, however, it should be noted that the response to the intake of food supplements may vary from woman to woman; for this reason, it is not possible to say that the intake of food supplements is always useful, in all women and in any situation. Once again, your doctor will tell you if they are a good idea for you.

What do food supplements contain?

The ingredients that can be included in the composition of food supplements are many.

Among these, we recall the following categories.

- **Vitamins**. Vitamins are perhaps the best known ingredients. According to the current legislation regarding these products, the following vitamins may be contained within them: vitamin A; vitamins of group B (B1, B2, niacin, pantothenic acid, B6, folic acid and B12); vitamin C; vitamin D; Vitamin E; vitamin K.

- **Minerals**. They are often associated with vitamins within the well-known dietary supplements of vitamins and minerals. The current regulations provide for the possibility of including the following minerals in the ingredients of these products: calcium; magnesium; iodine; iron; copper; zinc; manganese; sodium; potassium; selenium; chrome; molybdenum; silicon; boron; fluoride and chloride.

- **Amino acids.** Essential and branched amino acids can also be part of the composition of food supplements. Examples of amino acids that can be found in these products are valine, leucine, isoleucine, arginine, carnitine, cysteine, etc. However, please note that, in most cases, the amino acids mentioned above are found in the form of salts or derivatives and not in pure form.

- **Omega series fatty acids.** These are essential fatty acids. Food supplements contain mainly fatty acids of the omega-3 series in association or not with fatty acids of the omega-6 series. However, the lack of the latter is generally rare, which is why omega-3s are often preferred as supplement ingredients.

- **Prebiotics and probiotics**. They are used to promote and restore the normal balance of the intestinal bacterial flora which can be altered due to stress, taking drugs (antibiotics), etc.

- **Herbs, extracts and other herbal preparation.** The herbs and their derivatives that can be used in food supplements are really huge in number, varying according to the type of product that needs to be created. To cite a few examples, there are food supplements containing parts, extracts or derivatives of psyllium, ginkgo, blueberry, grape, valerian, ginseng, eleutherococcus, hawthorn, turmeric, ginger, etc.

- **Other active substances not included in the categories we just mentioned.** A well-known example is given by coenzyme Q10, but also by some types of enzymes (for example, bromelain), phytosterols, flavonoids, phospholipids, melatonin, etc.

Other ingredients or excipients

In addition to the substances described above, food supplements contain additional ingredients, also known as excipients. These are substances that are added to the final product for different purposes. Among these, we recall the following.

- **Substances that allow the maintenance of the characteristics of the supplement**. As mentioned, food supplements can be made in the form of tablets, effervescent tablets,

tablets, capsules, gummy candies, powders, liquids. To ensure that the supplements maintain shape, consistency, dilution, release of the active substances after ingestion or other chemical-physical characteristics, it is necessary to add particular substances to the formulation. For example, substances are usually added to tablets and capsules that allow them to be kept sufficiently compact in order to avoid crumbling by handling; substances are added to the effervescent tablets which allow them to be dissolved in water with effervescence, in fact; substances capable of maintaining the particular consistency can be added to the gummy candies as well and so on.

- **Dyes**. They are used to give the product a captivating color in order to ensure a better visual appearance. Of course, food dyes are used.

- **Coating agents**. They are used to give the surface of the product a uniform, smooth and sometimes shiny appearance.

- **Flavors**. Used to give the product a pleasant flavor.

- **Preservatives and antioxidants.** Used to ensure optimal conservation and non-degradation of the product.

Side effects

In the vast majority of cases, food supplements are well tolerated and, generally, are not responsible for the onset of particular side effects. However, this occurrence cannot be excluded with absolute certainty and, in some cases, it is still possible to encounter the appearance of undesirable effects. The type and intensity of side effects that could potentially occur can vary depending on several factors, such as the following.

- The type of supplement taken and the type of ingredients it contains;
- The presence of any problems, disorders and diseases affecting different organs and tissues, their type and their degree of severity;

- The frequency of taking food supplements and the amount of product taken (Note: it is important to respect the dosage indicated on the package / package leaflet and any doctor's instructions).

Finally, it should be remembered that even the onset of any allergic reactions in sensitive women cannot be ruled out. These reactions can be triggered both by the active substances and by the excipients contained in food supplements.

Side effects and natural food supplements

Many people are led to believe that taking food supplements based on natural products or extracts (for example, medicinal plants) is completely harmless and safe. However, this belief - in addition to being unfounded - could even prove to be dangerous. In fact, it is very important to specify that "natural" is not synonymous with "safe"; therefore, it is necessary to always pay the utmost caution even in the consumption of natural food supplements, even more so if you are pregnant, breastfeeding or if you suffer from ailments, problems or diseases of any kind. On the other hand, it is also true that the active substances contained in food supplements are present in such quantities that - with correct use and respecting the dosage - they should not cause any harm. Despite this, in the presence of particular conditions - such as, for example, allergies and diseases - even a small amount of a given substance can give rise to serious side effects.

Contraindications of food supplements
The main contraindication to the use of food supplements concerns the presence of known allergies to the active substances and / or to one or more of the excipients (flavors, dyes, preservatives, etc.) contained in the product.

In addition to this, the intake of some food supplements containing certain substances may be contraindicated during menopause, and in the presence of disorders and pathologies.

For example, women with heart or kidney disease should not take food supplements so lightly, as even substances that are considered harmless under normal and healthy conditions - such as, for example, some natural extracts, minerals, trace elements and amino acids - could be harmful and dangerous in the presence of pathological conditions. Clearly, given the large number of supplements in circulation and the equally large variety of ailments and pathologies that can contraindicate their use, it is difficult to estimate a complete and exhaustive list of all possible contraindications. Talk to your doctor before starting an intermittent fasting protocol and you will get more information about the right supplements for you as well.

Correct approach

To be able to approach food supplements correctly, it is first of all necessary to know these products, to know what they are, what they are for, for what purposes they were designed and when it is appropriate to use them. In this regard, it is important to underline the fact that, in general, the use of food supplements is advisable only if there is actually a need for them. A healthy woman, under normal conditions, who has no deficiencies of any kind and who adopts healthy intermittent fasting protocols, normally, should not need to resort to any type of dietary supplement.

At the same time, food supplements cannot be considered as the emergency remedy to be used in case of unregulated intermittent fasting protocols and lifestyles. Not surprisingly, on the packaging of these products there is always the phrase:

"Food supplements are not intended as a substitute for a varied and balanced diet and a correct lifestyle".

Let's take a practical example to better understand this concept. Taking so-called anti-aging food supplements - which are normally rich in antioxidants - to counteract skin damage caused by bad habits (such as, for example, smoking or uncontrolled exposure to UV rays) makes no sense, if in everyday life, the aforementioned wrong behaviors continue to be adopted. On the other hand, even if said habits are corrected, it is not certain that the aforementioned supplements prove to be really effective in improving the skin appearance.

For a correct use of food supplements, it is also important to remember that these products are not drugs and, therefore, are not able to cure any type of ailment or disease.

Rather, if the doctor deems it useful and necessary, in the presence of particular health problems or diseases, he can prescribe the intake of supplements as an extra "treatment" to traditional therapeutic strategies.

Another particularly important point is that concerning posology. The quantity of food supplement taken and the duration of the "treatment" - shown on the package or on the package leaflet or expressly indicated by the doctor - must be strictly respected. Even if the supplements are not medicines, in fact, it is always and in any case necessary to follow the recommended doses.

Summarizing what has been said so far, we could say that the correct approach for the right use of food supplements cannot be separated from the knowledge of the following basic concepts.

- Food supplements are not drugs.
- Food supplements are not an alternative to a balanced diet and correct lifestyle habits.
- The use of food supplements does not improve a pre-existing state of health.
- The non-use of food supplements does not compromise or worsen the health of the individual.
- Food supplements are not dietary products. In other words, they are not products intended for a particular diet.
- The recommended dosage must always be respected.
- In the presence of diseases or other conditions (for example, particular allergies and menopause), it is necessary to seek medical advice before taking food supplements of any kind.

Now that we have discussed the basics concepts regarding supplements, it is time to dive deeper into those that are actually recommended when following an intermittent fasting protocol.

Chapter 24

Choosing the Right Multivitamin for Your Intermittent Fasting Protocol

There are several reasons why women need to take multivitamins when following an intermittent fasting protocol. They are especially important for those who are in menopause or trying to get pregnant, as they offer additional help in supporting the body during these important events. Other women, on the other hand, have to take them to combat a particular deficiency. However, for most female subjects who are in good health, the best way to get vitamins is to eat a healthy diet, rich in fruits and vegetables.

Check with your doctor to find out if you have vitamin deficiencies

Many women think they are not deficient in vitamins, when in fact it may be insufficient to some extent. Normal blood tests do not detect the presence of these essential nutrients nor can they identify the levels of vitamin D produced by the body. Therefore, it is necessary to undergo more specific investigations to make sure that any deficiencies are discovered. In these cases, your doctor can help you develop a meal plan and possibly recommend the vitamins that suit your needs. Your doctor will likely recommend that you take them in the following cases.

- You typically consume less than 1600 calories per day.
- You follow an intermittent fasting protocol that does not contain sufficient amounts of fruits and vegetables. In this case, you should eat 90-180g of fruit and also add 300-450g of vegetables per day.
- You don't eat two or three servings of fish a week. In this case, your doctor may recommend fish oil supplements.

- You have a fairly heavy menstrual cycle: you may be subject to an iron deficiency.
- You have digestive problems that do not allow you to assimilate a sufficient amount of nutrients, while following a healthy diet.

Tell your doctor if you are a vegetarian or vegan

These eating habits tend to be indicated when you want to keep fat consumption and cholesterol levels low even during times when you are not following an intermittent fasting protocol. They are often associated with a lower risk of heart disease, high blood pressure, obesity and type 2 diabetes. However, it is important to make sure you are getting all the proteins, vitamins and minerals your body needs. If not, you may have deficiciens like the following ones.

- **Iron**. Many vegetarians have lower iron reserves than those who are omnivores. Consult your doctor to find out if your iron levels are low.

- **Vitamin B12**. Vegetarians can get it through the consumption of dairy products and eggs, but vegans must take supplements or eat foods enriched with vitamin B12. Read the nutritional values found on soy and rice milk products, on the packaging of breakfast cereals and meat substitutes.

- **Calcium**. Since meat and dairy products are high in calcium, many vegans are particularly prone to low calcium intake. This mineral is essential for maintaining bone health and avoiding fractures. If you are vegan, try to consume calcium-fortified foods, such as fruit juices, cereals, soy, and rice milk. This information is usually shown on the packaging. Also, you should check with your doctor to find out if you need to take calcium supplements.

- **Vitamin D**. The body produces vitamin D when it is exposed to the sun. However, the quantities it manages to synthesize depend on the use of sunscreen, the time of the day, the period of the year, the latitude and the pigmentation of the skin. Vitamin D is important for bone health. If you are concerned that you are not producing enough, consult your healthcare provider to find out if you should take supplements and eat foods enriched with this nutrient, including cow's milk, rice milk, soy milk, orange juice, cereals and margarine.

- **Zinc**. Soy, legumes, grains, cheese and nuts are excellent plant sources of zinc. If your diet is low in these foods, consult your doctor about possible solutions.

- **Long chain omega-3 fatty acids**. They are necessary to preserve eye health and the proper functioning of the brain. Many people get them by eating fish and eggs. If you don't consume these foods, you can also get them through flaxseed, canola oil, walnuts, soybeans, omega-3 fatty acid-enriched bars, or microalgae supplements. Ask your doctor if you need to assimilate them by consuming supplements.

Consider your age.

Postmenopausal women need to be careful about getting sufficient amounts of calcium and vitamin D to prevent osteoporosis. It is an important recommendation especially for older women who, living alone, run the risk of falling and suffering bone fractures. Female subjects over 50 should take the following amount of minerals.

- **800 IU (international units) of vitamin D per day**. Even exposure to the sun allows the body to produce it. Try to get out of the house and take a walk every day to make sure you get some sunlight.

- **1200 mg of calcium per day**. It is an important mineral that allows you to keep your bones strong and protect them from natural deterioration due to body movements.

Consult your doctor about taking vitamins in the prenatal period

If you are trying to conceive a child, are pregnant or breastfeeding, your doctor will likely recommend that you take a prenatal vitamin supplement. It is not a substitute for healthy nutrition, but it can help the fetus get all the nutrients it needs. These vitamins are specially designed for pregnant or breastfeeding women. You should not take them if you are not yet pregnant or if you are not breastfeeding. Prenatal vitamins typically contain the following ingredients.

- **Folic acid.** If you are trying to conceive or are pregnant, you need 600-800 mcg (micrograms) of folic acid per day. It promotes brain development in the early stages of fetal development. However, an overdose could hinder the detection of a possible vitamin B12 deficiency.

- **Iron**. If you are pregnant, you need about 27 mg (milligrams) of iron per day. If you take too much, you risk getting sick and suffering from constipation, vomiting, diarrhea or even life-threatening consequences.

- **Calcium**. It is a vital mineral for pregnant women because it promotes healthy bone development. Pregnant women should take

1000 mg per day. However, most prenatal vitamins only contain 200-300 mg. This means that you have to supplement the calcium requirement. You can get it by eating vegetables, such as broccoli, spinach, kale, turnips, savoy cabbage. Also consider other foods that contain added calcium, such as soy milk and fruit juices. In excessive amounts, it can increase the risk of kidney stones.

- **Vitamin D**. If you are pregnant, you should be getting sufficient amounts of vitamin D to support the baby's bone health. The Mayo Clinic (a non-profit organization for medical practice and research in the United States) recommends 600 IU (international units) of vitamin D per day. You can reach this amount by exposing yourself to the sun and consuming fish (especially fatty ones like salmon), fruit juices with added vitamin D, milk and eggs.

Ask your doctor if vitamin supplements can interfere with the action of medications

Some vitamins can interact with the way the body metabolizes drugs. If you are on medication, ask your doctor or dietician about vitamin supplements before you start taking them to make sure you are safe. Here's what some supplements do to the body.

- Vitamin D can affect blood glucose and blood pressure, but also interact with birth control pills and drug treatments for HIV, asthma, cancer, heart disease, cholesterol problems, pain relievers and other medications.

- Vitamin B6 can increase the risk of bleeding if it interacts with aspirin or other blood thinners. If you are diabetic, ask your doctor about taking vitamin B6 before taking it, as it can affect the blood sugar level. It can also negatively interact with medications for asthma, cancer, depression, Parkinson's disease, and other conditions.

- Vitamin E can also increase the risk of bleeding when taken in combination with blood thinners. It could also affect the action of drugs against Alzheimer's disease, tuberculosis, cancer, asthma, heart disease, seizures and other diseases.

- Vitamin C can interfere with anticoagulants and affect blood glucose and blood pressure, but also interact with oral birth control pills, HIV medications, acetaminophen, Parkinson's disease medicines, antibiotics, anticancer drugs, aspirin, barbiturates, and other substances.

As you can see, it is important to talk to your doctor before taking any supplement.

Consider a multivitamin

The advantage of multivitamins is that most of them are designed to offer the recommended daily allowance (RDA) of different vitamins and minerals. The RDA should be sufficient - therefore, not contraindicated - for most women in good health.

Look at the labels on the products

You should find a table that tells you what percentage of each individual nutrient is contained in the product based on the RDA. The best proportions provide about 100% of the daily requirement of different vitamins and minerals.

If your doctor thinks it helps, you can buy a multivitamin at a drugstore.

Do not take excessive doses of any particular vitamin

If the label on the package indicates that it provides much more than 100% of the recommended daily allowance, then that is what is known as a megadose. For example, 500% of the RDA of a certain mineral is a megadose. In fact, excessive intake of some vitamins can be harmful and have the following consequences.

- Too high or too low amounts of vitamin B6 can cause problems to the nervous system.

- It is easier to experience an overdose of fat-soluble vitamins (A, D, E, K) rather than water-soluble vitamins, as the excess is not excreted in the urine. For example, too much vitamin A can increase the risk of hip fracture, while too much vitamin D can promote exorbitant amounts of calcium in the blood and cause vomiting and constipation.

- Excessive iron intake can cause vomiting and liver damage.

- Vitamins and minerals are often added to industrial foods and drinks. If your intermittent fasting protocol favors a large supply of certain vitamins, be aware that you may need to reduce your supplement intake since you are already getting the right amounts of these nutrients.

Don't take expired vitamins

Vitamins can degrade over time. This deterioration is more likely especially if you store them in warm, humid places. If they have expired, it is safer and healthier to buy them again. If you're considering taking certain vitamins that don't have an expiration date, don't take them.

Research the vitamins you are considering

The content of vitamins and supplements available on the market is not subject to strict quality control as is the case with food. This means that it is difficult to know exactly what these pills contain.

Check if the supplements you intend to take are present in the special register made available by the Ministry of Health.

Get adequate amounts of folic acid

Women who are not pregnant need 400 mcg of folic acid, or folate, per day. It is a vitamin belonging to group B, which is important for the nervous system. Excellent sources of folic acid include the following foods.

- Whole grains or grains enriched with folic acid
- Spinach;
- Beans;
- Asparagus;
- Oranges;
- Peanuts.

Eat foods rich in iron

The body better assimilates iron from meat, especially red meat. However, if you are a vegetarian, you can still meet your iron needs by increasing the consumption of foods that are rich in iron, even if they are not of animal origin. Before menopause, women should take 18 mg per day. After menopause, the daily intake drops to 8 mg. Excellent sources of iron include the following foods.

Red meat (lean meat is healthier, because it contains less fat);

- Pork;
- White meat;
- Seafood;
- Beans
- Peas;
- Spinach;
- Raisins and dehydrated apricots;
- Foods that contain added iron, such as cereals, breads, and pasta. On the package you will find written if they have been enriched or not.

Calculate if you are getting enough calcium

After menopause, women's daily calcium requirement increases from 1000 mg to 1200 mg per day. It is important to take it in sufficient quantities to prevent osteoporosis. A calcium deficiency can be avoided by consuming the following foods.

- Milk;
- Yogurt;
- Cheese;
- Broccoli;
- Spinach;
- Kale
- Turnips;
- Cabbage;
- Calcium-enriched soy milk and fruit juices;
- Salmon.

Get sufficient amounts of vitamin B6

It is an essential nutrient for the proper functioning of the nervous system. It is rare to suffer from a deficiency, but it is possible to completely avoid this possibility by consuming these foods.

- Cereals;

- Carrots;
- Peas;
- Spinach;
- Milk;
- Cheese;
- Eggs;
- Fish;
- Flour.

Get out in the sun to take enough vitamin D

When exposing to sunlight, don't forget to use sunscreen to avoid sunburn. The recommended amount for women is 600 IU (international units) per day. For women over 50, on the other hand, an additional intake of 200 IU per day is recommended. It is important because it promotes bone strength when, at a certain age, the risk of bone fractures is higher than in younger women. Vitamin D can also be obtained by consuming the following foods.

- Milk;
- Yogurt;
- Salmon;
- Trout;

- Tuna fish;
- Halibut.

Eat carrots to get vitamin A

This vitamin is important for the visual system, cell growth and proper functioning of the immune system. In adequate quantities, it can also help prevent cancer. You can get it by consuming the following foods.

- Yellow vegetables;
- Liver;
- Kidneys;
- Eggs and dairy products.

Cook with an oil that guarantees a sufficient supply of vitamin E

In addition to eggs, cereals enriched with this vitamin, fruit, spinach, red and white meat and nuts, it is contained in many qualities of oil, including the following ones.

- Corn oil;
- Cottonseed oil;
- Safflower oil;
- Soybean oil;

- Sunflower oil;
- Argan oil;
- Olive oil;
- Wheat germ oil.

Protect the health of the circulatory system with vitamin K

Vitamin K is necessary for the blood because it promotes blood clotting. You can get it in sufficient quantities by eating the following foods.

- Green leafy vegetables
- Meat;
- Dairy product.

Chapter 25

Vitamin C and Vitamin D: Your Best Friends During Intermittent Fasting

Vitamin C and Vitamin D are two of the most important vitamins to assume during an intermittent fasting protocol. In fact, as we have seen in the previous chapters, vitamins can have a profound impact on the result of an intermittent fasting protocol.

In the next few pages we are diving deeper into this topic, trying to highlight the most important factors that make these two vitamins an incredible asset during your diet.

Vitamin C, also called ascorbic acid, is a water-soluble antioxidant that helps keep infections under control, neutralize free radicals, and promote iron absorption. It also helps produce collagen, which is essential for the health of teeth, organs, bones and blood vessels. Unlike most animals, humans do not have the ability to independently produce vitamin C, so it is necessary to assimilate it every day, constantly. Any food containing at least 10% per serving of the recommended daily intake can be considered a good source of vitamin C. The good news is that vitamin C is found in many healthy foods, so for those looking to increase their consumption, it won't be hard to do so.

Vitamin C is essential for memory, helps prevent cell mutations, premature aging and oxidation of fatty foods, and also strengthens the immune system.
Some believe that vitamin C cures or stops the common cold, but there is no convincing scientific evidence for it. However, by strengthening the immune system, it is possible that vitamin C protects the body from pathogens that cause colds, so it may relieve it and perhaps shorten its duration, but it will hardly prevent it. Please be aware of online scammers

that tell you that vitamin C is the solution to every health problem, it is simply not true.

Relationship between diet and vitamin C consumption

Most people should be able to get adequate amounts of vitamin C by following a healthy, nutrient-rich intermittent fasting protocol. If you eat junk food, you are unlikely to get a good dose of vitamin C from your intermittent fasting protocol. However, it is enough to change one's eating habits to increase the assimilation of ascorbic acid.

Since vitamin C neutralizes some food inhibitors, such as phytates (found in whole grains) and tannins (found in tea and coffee), increasing your intake of vitamin C can help optimize nutrition and lead a healthier lifestyle.

Relationship between vitamin C and stress

A vitamin C depletion can cause stress. If the tension is constant, it will soon drain all vitamin C stores. Eating foods rich in ascorbic acid or taking supplements when you feel stressed can have a positive effect on your diet and well-being. If you are aware of what you eat and the micronutrients of each food, you can adjust your intermittent fasting protocol to make sure you are getting enough vitamin C.

Symptoms that tend to characterize a possible vitamin C deficiency

When you have health problems, you should always go to a doctor directly to be on the safe side, but the following symptoms may be associated with a vitamin C deficiency: gums, scarring problems and reduced immune defenses against infections. These symptoms are not necessarily indicative of a vitamin C deficiency, but you can speak to your doctor in case you are concerned.

Acute vitamin C deficiency can cause a condition called scurvy, which occurs when the body cannot produce collagen or absorb iron due to vitamin C deficiency.

Few people in developed countries suffer from severe deficiencies. However, if you exclude vitamin C from your intermittent fasting protocol for about 4 weeks, the deficiency can arise rather quickly.

People at particular risk include the elderly, drug users, alcoholics, individuals with mental illnesses, neglected dependents, individuals suffering from eating disorders such as anorexia or bulimia, smokers (they need more vitamin C to cope with the additional stress exerted on the organism) and individuals who tend to have difficult tastes when it comes to eating fruits and vegetables.

Remember that you need to take vitamin C every day. Vitamin C does not remain in the body, it must be constantly replenished. Eating a certain amount of citrus fruits on a given day only serves to temporarily satisfy the consumption of vitamin C. In fact the next day you will have to renew your supplies. It is estimated that women need a minimum of 45 mg of vitamin C per day. The optimal amounts are 90 mg for men, 75 mg for women and male adolescents, 65 mg for female adolescents. Pregnant or breastfeeding women need 75-120 mg per day.
Usually, if doses of vitamin C that exceed the recommended daily intake are taken, the excesses are expelled. In high doses it is not considered toxic, but it increases iron absorption, which can be a problem for

those suffering from hemochromatosis (excessive accumulation of iron in the body). Consequently, if you are already eating a balanced diet, it is not necessary to take vitamin C supplements.

Additionally, overdoing vitamin C can cause abdominal pain, nausea, headaches, fatigue, kidney stones, and diarrhea.

Get enough vitamin C during your meals

This is essential to reap all the benefits. Vitamin C supplements are measured in milligrams. Many foods contain it, so consuming them can help you increase your ascorbic acid intake.

Pineapple contains 16 mg of vitamin C, asparagus 31 mg, raw broccoli 89 mg, dried tomatoes in oil 101 mg, raw parsley 133 mg. Apples are so rich in phytonutrients that a single serving has antioxidant properties equivalent to 1000 mg of vitamin C.

Citrus fruits are a particularly rich source of vitamin C. For example, 230g of grapefruit is enough to meet your daily requirement of vitamin C, while a glass of orange juice is equivalent to 165% of your daily intake of vitamin C. Fresh orange juice or an orange is preferable to a packaged juice.

Furthermore, the vitamin C contained in citrus fruits helps fight stress because it lowers the levels of the stress hormone and reduces blood pressure, increases the energy level by promoting iron absorption and provides other essential phytonutrients that work in synergy with the ascorbic acid (some of them improve memory).

Pay attention to the recommended doses of vitamin C we mentioned
Consult the nutrition table prepared by the Health Ministry and look for the recommended doses. You will be surprised to find that it is really easy to vary your intermittent fasting protocol in order to include enough sources of vitamin C.

Pay attention to the shelf life of your vitamin C sources. It is not convenient to store them for a long time, in fact over time they will lose their properties. As a result, try to eat foods that are as fresh as possible rather than leaving them in the refrigerator or pantry. For example, if you leave broccoli in the fridge and then boil it, the vitamin C content will drop considerably, while freshly steamed broccoli has much more.

If possible, grow vegetables indoors, just grow broccoli on the balcony and potatoes in a sack or barrel.

Wash the fruit and vegetables, then let them dry. Store them in an airtight container in the fridge and eat them within a few days. Do not immerse or store them in water, otherwise the vitamin C will dissolve in the liquid. It also disperses in the cooking water.

Fresh foods are the best sources of vitamin C, which is found in most fruits and vegetables. In particular, try to eat foods from the cabbage family, red and green peppers, potatoes, black currants, strawberries, citrus fruits, and tomatoes.

Eat lots of green leafy vegetables [27], including broccoli, kale, Brussels sprouts, and spinach, raw or steamed. Use only a small amount of water to maximize the vitamin content.

Go for a spinach-based salad rather than a lettuce-based one. Raw spinach contains more vitamin C. To fill up on ascorbic acid, enrich your salad with tomatoes, green and red peppers. Vegetables lose micronutrients with cooking.

Incorporate more potatoes into your diet

They are another great source of Vitamin C. You may have heard that Vitamin C is concentrated in the peel, but it is not ture, although it has other benefits. For example, the peel is rich in fiber. When baking potatoes, be sure to eat the peel as well.

Vitamin B and juices

If you count fruit juice when you calculate your daily vitamin C intake, pay attention. The juice contains a lot of calories, not to mention that it does not have the properties of the actual fruit. To increase your consumption of vitamin C, you should make the juice with the pulp, because vitamin C is better absorbed when combined with bioflavonoids, which are found mainly in the pulp.

Drink some fresh juice

Make it at home or buy frozen concentrates and avoid the packaged juices you find in the fridge. Frozen concentrates have significantly higher doses of vitamin

C. In fact, the pasteurization process that characterizes industrially produced juices partially eliminates vitamin C.

Vitamin C and supplements

Take vitamin C supplements in tablet form. There are a number of over-the-counter supplement brands. They have different dosages: you should take the one that best suits your needs. If you are unsure, ask your pharmacist for advice.

Use a topical supplement. Vitamin C preparations for local use are good for the skin. Studies have been carried out to evaluate their rejuvenating effect on mature or wrinkled skin.

Use chewable vitamin C tablets. There are supplements in tablet form that taste amazing. They should be chewed well and then ingested.

Use soluble vitamin C tablets, another product to supplement ascorbic acid which usually tastes pretty good. Let the tablet dissolve completely on your tongue. It is recommended not to eat, drink or smoke during this process. It is quite effective when you feel a bit sick, because vitamin C has a positive effect on energy levels and the immune system.

Now that we have discussed the incredible power of vitamin C, it is time to dive deeper into another great vitamin that you should include in your intermittent fasting protocol. We are talking about vitamin D and the next few pages are going to tell you more about it.

Vitamin D is a nutrient that can prevent several chronic diseases, including some cancers. However, many women lack it because most foods don't contain enough of it. In fact, the richest source of vitamin D is the sun, but being exposed to sunlight for too long is dangerous for the skin. It is not easy to satisfy your daily needs for this nutrient, but thanks to an adequate intermittent fasting protocol, careful exposure to the sun and taking supplements, you can get the benefits of this precious element.

Take supplements

Although it is important for health, this vitamin is not present in sufficient quantities in foods, therefore it is not possible to assimilate an adequate dose simply with a healthy intermittent fasting protocol. While you can look for foods that are particularly rich in it, supplements are an important aspect of improving health and increasing this rare resource. You can find vitamin D supplements in two forms: vitamin D2 (ergocalciferol) and vitamin D3 (cholecalciferol).

Vitamin D3 occurs naturally in fish and is processed by the body when it metabolizes sunlight. It is also believed to be less toxic, in large quantities, than vitamin D2, although it is a more potent form and offers greater health benefits.

Most experts recommend vitamin D3 over D2. Ask your doctor for advice on the dosage and quality of the various brands.

Be sure to take magnesium supplements as well. This other element is needed to absorb vitamin D, but is completely depleted during this process. If you only take vitamin D without supplementing magnesium, you can suffer from a deficiency of that mineral.

Choose vitamin D2 supplements if you are vegan. Vitamin D3 is more complete, but it is of animal origin. Therefore, if you are vegan or vegetarian, you will avoid these types of products, regardless of the health benefits. Vitamin D2, on the other hand, is synthetically produced using molds and does not contain products of animal origin.

Increase your sun exposure while still protecting your skin

Although vitamin D is scarce in foods, it is abundant in sunlight. It is important to find the right balance between too much and too little exposure, because you don't have to risk getting burned. To find a good solution, you can spend 10-20 minutes in the sun twice a week, putting sunscreen only on your face. Alternatively, you can spend 2-3 minutes in the sun several times a week, always putting the protection on your face only. Either way, make sure you don't bathe for an hour after being in the sun. Your body needs some time to absorb the vitamin it has produced.

Be careful not to over-expose yourself to UV rays, as they can cause skin cancer. In the United States, 1.5 million cases are recorded each year. Avoid getting burned in the sun, not so much because of the pain, but because it causes damage to skin cells that can cause abnormal and cancerous growth.

Continue to use sunscreen on any other occasions you expose yourself to the sun. You will likely be able to absorb vitamin D even with sunscreen, but its ability to protect the skin from harmful UV rays also limits the production of vitamin D.

Your skin does not need to tan to be able to absorb vitamin D from the sun.

Learn about the factors that can affect sun-triggered vitamin D production

An important factor is the proximity to the equator. In fact, people who live in this geographic area inevitably have more opportunities to expose themselves to the sun than those who live in areas further north or south. The natural color of the skin also affects the ability to absorb vitamin D; individuals with a lighter skin produce it more quickly than those with a darker skin tone, due to the melanin content.

Even if you can't intervene on these factors, you can still choose the time of day to go outside and get sunlight. It is best to expose yourself during the central hours of the day, rather than early in the morning or in the evening, because at this stage of the day the sun is stronger and the body produces more vitamin D.

Expose as much skin as possible to the sun. During these few minutes that you are purposely in the sun, you should not cover your body with long-sleeved trousers or clothing. The more skin is exposed to the sun, the more vitamin D is synthesized. However, use common sense; if you live in an area where the sun is very strong, by respecting this advice you risk getting burned.

Keep in mind that sun exposure is very high even on a completely cloudy day

The body is able to store vitamin D, so if you stay out in the sun systematically in spring or summer, you will have enough for the whole year.

Eat foods rich in vitamin D

While you can't get enough of this element on a normal intermittent fasting protocol, you can still try to get as much of it from foods as possible. The richest natural source is fish, such as salmon, mackerel, tuna and sardines. If you are brave enough you can also try cod liver oil. Dairy products, egg yolk and cheese also contain small amounts of vitamin D.

Look for fortified products. As awareness of the benefits of vitamin D increases, so does the number of food companies that enrich their products with this vitamin. Read the nutrition information label to find out if a product has been enriched. Among the most common are milk and breakfast cereals.

Limit your caffeine intake
Studies have found that it interferes with vitamin D receptors and inhibits their absorption. Due to its effects on vitamin D, caffeine also negatively affects calcium levels in the body, since one function of vitamin D is to promote its absorption. Avoid drinking too many drinks containing this substance, such as coffee, tea, and other caffeinated sodas.

As you might have understood by now, there is not a single thing you can do to ensure adequate levels of vitamin D. Studies have found that supplements are not as effective a source of nutrients as food, but it is also true that foods do not provide enough vitamin D for optimal health. The only abundant natural source of this nutrient - the sun - is also very dangerous when exposure is excessive and can cause cancer. The best approach to increasing vitamin D levels is to combine all three methods: supplements, sunlight, and nutrition.

Benefits of vitamin D

Many studies have shown that vitamin D is very effective as a means of preventing numerous chronic diseases. In particular, it is able to increase the body's ability to absorb calcium, preventing bone problems such as rickets, osteomalacia (softening of the bones) and osteoporosis. Other research suggests that increasing the intake of vitamin D can lower blood pressure, reduce the chances of heart attack and stroke, develop autoimmune diseases, such as rheumatoid arthritis, and multiple sclerosis.

Dangers of a vitamin D deficiency

It is important to put in place all possible techniques to increase the levels of this vitamin in the body, because its deficiency is related to a number of chronic diseases. Hypovitaminosis D is linked to type 1 diabetes, chronic pain - both muscle and bone - and several types of cancers, including colon, breast, prostate, ovary, esophagus, and lymphatic system.

About 40-75% of the population is deficient in vitamin D, mainly because this nutrient is not abundant in natural food sources and many people live in areas where it is not possible to get enough exposure to the sun. Increased awareness of the correlation between UV rays and skin cancer has increased the use of sunscreens, which lower the production of vitamin D.

Although 40-75% of the population does not meet their vitamin D needs, there are some categories that are more likely to be deficient in this nutrient. You must be aware of these factors in order to act accordingly and monitor your vitamin D levels.

The risk categories are the following.
- Women suffering from photodermatitis for whom sunlight is toxic;
- Women who rarely go outside;
- Women suffering from heliophobia;

- Malnourished women who develop extreme sensitivity to light;
- Women suffering from malabsorption diseases;
- Those women who wear clothes every day that cover them from head to toe;
- The elderly, whose absorption capacity by the skin is lower;
- Women who stay inside buildings all day, for example those who work in shopping centers;
- Women who follow a very strict intermittent fasting protocol without proper knowledge.

Getting tested for hypovitaminosis

See your doctor for a blood test called a 25 (OH) vitamin D test, or calcidiol. Your doctor will take a blood sample from you which will be analyzed in the laboratory.

If the doctor does not want to prescribe a blood test or you prefer another method, you can buy "do it yourself" tests on the internet. They are not very expensive (around 50 dollars) and can be a valid alternative.

It is not always easy to diagnose vitamin D deficiency, because its symptoms are similar to those of many other conditions. For this reason it is essential to check the levels regularly.

When you collect your calcidiol test results you will be able to understand them and change your intermittent fasting protocol based on them. Usually the value is expressed in ng/ml (nanograms per milliliter) or in nmol/l (nanomoles per liter). This indicates the amount of calcidiol in the blood, which in turn is a good reference for understanding the level of vitamin D.

According to the Endocrine Society, if your values are below 20 ng/mL (50 nmol/L), then you are vitamin D deficient. A result of 21-29 ng/mL (52.5–72.5 nmol/L) indicates some nutrient deficiency, but not a severe deficiency.

If your values fall within a deficiency or deficiency range, then make changes to your diet, get out in the sun and take supplements to increase your vitamin D intake.

Some women are better off when they have an amount of vitamin D that hovers around its recommended maximum levels. Find the amount that makes you feel good and keep it in check with supplements and foods rich in vitamin D.

If you follow these tips, you can be sure you will not have issues related to the deficiency of these two important vitamins. We highly recommend you plan ahead your vitamin intake before starting an intermittent fasting protocol.

Chapter 26

How to Stop Eating Processed Food

We want to dedicate the last chapter of this book to a very important topic. In fact, every intermittent fasting protocol is deemed to fail if you eat processed and unhealthy foods during your meals.

Most women over 50 are used to eating huge amounts of processed foods and this can have negative consequences when it comes to their health. By following the tips and tricks we share with you in this chapter, you are going to be able to improve the quality of your intermittent fasting protocol and conquer a healthier lifestyle.

Industrially processed foods have a bad reputation. They are very often associated with a high calorie content, with added fats and sugars, they are poor from a nutritional point of view and rich instead of chemicals and preservatives. However, the definition of junk food is currently quite broad and includes many different foods. In general, processed food means any food that has been deliberately processed before being eaten. When trying to reduce their consumption, it is important to consider the level of industrial processing. Highly refined, pre-cooked foods, rich in sugar, flavorings, dyes, preservatives or additives to improve texture are typical examples of the foods you should limit or exclude from your intermittent fasting protocol. By cutting out or cutting down on highly processed foods, you can eat healthier and more nutritious. In the following pages we are going to give you some tips to reduce the consumption of these foods.

Keep track of your meals

When trying to eliminate certain foods or food groups from your intermittent fasting protocol, it can help to keep a journal where you can write down your habits.

This way, you will be more aware of what processed foods you are eating, when you eat them, and how often.

Buy a diary or download an application on your smartphone. The ideal would be to write down the meals of a few working days and a few weekends. You may find that you eat differently on weekends than on weekdays, even if following your intermittent fasting protocol with precision.

Many times, people choose industrially processed foods for convenience. They are late for work, do not have time to cook, or have no other choice available when they are hungry. Pay attention to your eating habits: maybe you are always late in the morning and end up buying breakfast at fast food, without even getting out of the car.

It can help you to gradually eliminate industrial foods from your diet. As you rule out certain foods, you can replace them with less processed, more natural foods. By noting on paper what you need to eat, you can visually organize the meals for the whole week.

During your free moments, invest time to write down different meal and snack ideas. These notes can also become the basis for the shopping list.

When drafting your personal intermittent fasting protocol, be sure to take into account the amount of "on the fly" meals you need to eat during the week. By planning them in advance, you will be less tempted to take industrial foods.

Clean up the kitchen

Before re-evaluating your intermittent fasting protocol, think about what you typically buy at the grocery store and what you keep in the kitchen. Look in the refrigerator, freezer and pantry for processed foods, so free yourself from any temptation.

The items you need to check include the following.

- sweets such as ice cream, candies, cookies and snacks;
- potato chips, crackers, or pretzels;
- breakfast cereals, sauces, dressings or marinades;
- meats and cheeses;
- frozen appetizers or pre-cooked meals ready to be heated in the microwave.

These are typically all high in preservatives and high in sodium, something you want to limit while intermittent fasting.

Since almost all foods go through a process, decide which ones you want to eliminate and which ones to keep. For example, canned beans are processed, but they are also an excellent source of fiber and protein. Also, as long as you rinse them and throw away the storage liquid, they are considered low in sodium. This is a food that you should consider keeping in your intermittent fasting protocol.

The other processed foods you can keep are the following.

- canned vegetables with no added salt and low in sodium;
- whole grain foods (such as wholemeal pasta or rice);
- pre-washed and chopped vegetables (like ready-made salads in bags);
- totally natural nut butter.

If you don't feel like throwing away all this food, you can donate it to a charity or eat it in smaller doses until you change your intermittent fasting protocol and eat mostly natural foods.

Tips to avoid processed foods while shopping

When you go to the supermarket, you should forgo all processed snacks. Above all, go along the outermost and perimeter aisles, those in which the most wholemeal and natural foods are usually displayed. Try to choose products that come from these departments: fruit and vegetables, fresh meat and fish counter, shelves of dairy products and eggs.

Generally, the frozen food sector is also located around the perimeter of the supermarket and you can find both highly processed and almost natural foods. As long as the products don't contain too many sauces, toppings, and too many additives, they are still considered an acceptable and nutritious choice.

Be wary of the foods you find in the middle aisles. If you need to buy processed foods, choose only healthy and nutritious ones, such as canned beans, whole grains, and canned vegetables. Also make sure they don't contain too many added ingredients. For example, choose plain pasta instead of pasta with added flavorings or sauces, or low-sodium canned vegetables instead of those rich in seasonings or other flavorings.

If some of your favorite foods are in these aisles and you are tempted to buy them, completely avoid going near these shelves. For example, don't go to the area where the candy and chips are located, so you won't be tempted to put these products in your shopping cart.

Read the labels on all packaged foods. Since food processing can vary greatly, reading the labels gives you more details and accurate information about their process, what has been altered and what has been added.

The list of ingredients allows consumers to know exactly the content of the product. The label shows all the elements present in descending order, starting from the main ingredient to the one with the lowest dosage. In addition, you can check if the product contains additives, preservatives or other flavors.

There are several tips or tricks to help the consumer understand if the level of industrial processing is acceptable. Usually, it is advised not to buy those products that contain elements that are difficult to pronounce or incomprehensible. For example, some processed foods contain substances such as: diacetyl (a flavor of butter) or potassium sorbate (a chemical used to prolong shelf life). If you don't know what it means, you don't buy it.

Keep in mind that if a manufacturer brand has patented a proprietary blend (of ingredients such as spices or flavorings), it must indicate the ingredients, but not always the proportions. If the label shows this type of information, you shouldn't buy the product.
Be aware that some additives can make the product more nutritious. For example, some companies add vitamins or minerals to their foods. Even if these substances are unfamiliar to you, they actually improve the nutritional value of food.

Buy and eat fruits and vegetables. These are highly nutritious foods that contain essential substances, such as vitamins, minerals, fiber and antioxidants. At least half of each meal should consist of fruit or vegetables.

Agricultural products that have undergone minimal industrial treatment and which you should focus on are the following.

- fresh fruits and vegetables such as bananas, apples, tomatoes, aubergines;
- pre-cut and washed products, such as salad in bags or pre-cooked steamed green beans;

From canned foods, choose those low in sodium and with no added salt, prepared without sauces or other condiments.

Avoid over-processed products, such as fruit in syrup or sweetened, frozen or canned vegetables rich in sauces or other condiments.

Buy and eat very little processed protein. These are essential nutrients for a healthy diet, and meat is a great source of high-quality protein to add to your diet. You should often include some protein in your meals or snacks.

Among the little industrially processed protein foods are: poultry, red meat, pork, eggs and dairy products. Choose products of organic origin if you want to avoid those that contain hormones or preservatives.

The proteins of vegetable origin that have undergone minimal treatment are: dried beans, lentils, even canned peas (as long as without added salt or in any case by rinsing and throwing the preservation liquid), frozen legumes without the addition of sauces or condiments. Tofu, tempeh, and seitan are plant-based proteins, but are generally considered more processed.

Among the partially industrially processed protein sources are: frozen meat without the addition of additives and sauces, natural yogurt and cheeses.

The foods that have undergone a significant transformation and that you must avoid are: cured meats, hot dogs, sausages, bacon, pre-cooked and then frozen meat or ready-made meat-based meals.

Buy and eat lightly processed grains
Whole grains are the best choice, which are very high in fiber and nutrients. However, not all whole grains are free from industrial treatments, so be careful.
The less processed ones you should focus on the most are: raw brown rice, quinoa, millet, whole wheat couscous and barley. Wholemeal pasta has undergone

a major processing process, but it is a healthy supplement to your diet.

Do not buy precooked products, ready to heat in the microwave or that claim that can be cooked when in a hurry, because they have undergone further industrial processing to reduce preparation times at home.

You should also avoid refined grains such as rice, pasta and white bread, sweets, cakes and biscuits.

Once you have the right stock in the kitchen, you can start cooking your dishes without overly elaborate foods. Make sure that protein (poultry, red meat, pork, fish, low-fat dairy or legumes), fruits and vegetables form the basis of your meals.

An easy way to start cooking is to prepare the main course based on proteins. Add to this one or two ingredients, such as fruit, vegetables, or whole grains, to complete the meal.

Do not eat pre-made products such as prepackaged ones, frozen pizzas, pre-cooked meals, canned soups or pre-made sandwiches.

Have healthy snacks if allowed by your intermittent fasting protocol.

If you're hungry between meals, it's time for a snack. If you don't have a natural snack on hand, you'll be tempted to buy packaged ones, which are quick and easy. You should originally prepare healthy snacks to take with you at all times, to avoid overeating the industrially processed ones.

Try to have as many natural and healthy snacks with you as possible, if they are permitted by your intermittent fasting protocol. For example, have some fruit on hand (like apples), dried fruit or muesli prepared by yourself and take them to work. If you have the option to use a refrigerator, save certain foods, such as natural yogurt, raw vegetables, homemade hummus, or hard-boiled eggs.

Avoid typical processed snacks like candy, chips, crackers, snacks, packaged cake slices, single-serving cookies, or cereal / protein bars.

If you forget the snacks you made yourself at home or have no way to get them, at least look for the less processed snacks. For example, in many vending machines you will find packages of roasted peanuts or mixed nuts.

Don't go to fast food restaurants even on your cheat days

Many inexpensive or fast food restaurants offer a variety of highly processed foods. Although the menus have improved in recent years, it is still very difficult to find natural, whole and unprocessed foods.

Burgers, French fries, chicken nuggets, hot dogs, pizzas and other similar foods are just examples of food you usually find in cheap restaurants or fast food restaurants. Not only have these dishes undergone significant transformations, but if you eat them regularly they increase the risk of serious diseases, such as heart disease, hypertension and obesity.

If you still have to eat or choose fast food items, at least look for those products that are less processed and as natural as possible. For example, opt for a salad and grilled chicken, as they are the least processed ones you can order.

Eat processed foods in moderation. By eliminating or reducing processed foods from your diet you can control your weight and improve your overall health. However, an occasional snack or meal of processed products is allowed and should not cause serious adverse effects. Choose wisely and decide what "in moderation" really means to you.

If among your favorite foods there are some that have undergone an industrial process, you don't necessarily have to exclude them completely; for example, you can decide to eat them every Friday night or just once a month.

Remember that eliminating some industrial foods from your diet is still a great start. Ultimately, deciding how much or which processed food you want to exclude from your diet is essentially up to you.

Choose healthy alternatives

The most common processed foods are often also the tastiest. Think about what your favorites are (like sweets, pretzels, or crunchy biscuits) and consider if you can find a healthier alternative to replace them.

For example, if you want to eat something sweet after your meal, instead of choosing chocolate or ice cream, you can cut some fruit or eat plain yogurt with a little honey.

If you're craving something salty to munch on, grab a few carrots and bits of celery to eat with homemade hummus.

One of the most important tips we can give you is to prepare your favorite meals and snacks at home. In this way, you can keep track of what you eat without giving up good food.

Some easy ideas of snacks to have at home are: toppings, sauces or marinades, muesli or cereals, soups, stews and broths, baked foods such as muffins, cookies, granola bars, wholemeal bread or hummus.

If you wish, you can also prepare fast food-like meals at home. Homemade chicken nuggets and fries are definitely a better alternative than their restaurant versions.

Whatever you do, try to reduce the amount of processed food you have on a regulars basis and remember that a healthy intermittent fasting protocol prefers whole and natural foods.

Conclusion

e would like to thank you for making it to the end of this book. We have done our best to ensure that every information contained is useful and helps you in your weight loss journey.

We know how frustrating it could be to start an intermittent fasting protocol and feeling discouraged by the fact that results do not appear immediately. As we repeated throughout the book, the goal of intermittent fasting is to create a healthy lifestyle that can support you over the years, not just give you a rapid decrease in weight.

By following the tips shared in this book, you will certainly burn fat, lose weight and feel much better. However, as we do not know you in person, our final recommendation can only be the following one.

Before starting an intermittent fasting protocol talk to your doctor and find out whether intermittent fasting could be a good idea for you or not. Remember, never sacrifice your health to fit into that new skirt you just got.

Be healthy and your weight will adapt.

To your success!